Qigong for Beginners:

Three Full Workouts for Strength and Balance

Liam Machlin

Copyright © 2017 by Liam Machlin

www.lmtaichi.com

ALL RIGHTS RESERVED. This book contains material protected under International and Federal Copyright Laws and Treaties. Any unauthorized reprint or use of this material is prohibited. No part of this book may be reproduced or transmitted in any form or by any means, electronic or mechanical, including photocopying, recording, or by any information storage and retrieval system without express written permission from the author.

Qigong for Beginners: Three Full Workouts for Strength and Balance

Publisher: Create Space Independent Publishing Platform.
First Edition
Printed in the United States of America
ISBN 151418978X
1. Qigong - Health Aspects. 2. Qigong– History. 3. Tai Chi.

Printed and bound in the United States

To Olivia, Mia and Stella.

CONTENTS

Introduction 5

Chapter 1: China History 9

Chapter 2: Qigong Basics 17

Chapter 3: Stances, Breath and Mind. 41

Chapter 4: Morning Qigong 51

Chapter 5: Eight Pieces of Brocade 65

Chapter 6: 18 Form Tai Chi Qigong 77

Chapter 7: Qigong for Healthy Lifestyle 103

Glossary of Qigong Terms 113

Bibliography 117

Qigong Videos 121

Introduction

"A human being is a part of a whole, called by us a universe, a part limited in time and space. He experiences himself, his thoughts and feelings as something separated from the rest . . . a kind of optical delusion of his consciousness. This delusion is a kind of prison for us, restricting us to our personal desires and to affection for a few persons nearest to us. Our task must be to free ourselves from this prison by widening our circle of compassion to embrace all living creatures and the whole of nature in its beauty."

– Albert Einstein

"The journey of a thousand miles begins with one step."
- Laozi

About 2000 years ago there was a big flood throughout the Yellow River Valley in China. Many villages were destroyed and many people got sick. The Emperor sent his physician to find out why so many people were getting sick. The physician came back and reported to the Emperor that people are like water, when they are moving they are healthy. When they stop moving and become lazy and stagnant diseases start to appear. Another discovery the physician had was that while the people were getting sick the animals were doing fine. The cure for the stagnation, reasoned the doctor, was movement! The physician decided to create a system to teach people how to move like animals. The physician's name was Hua Tua and what he created was the Five Animal Frolics which is one of the oldest Qigong exercises and still practiced today. What Hua Tua had observed was that the energy in our body- the Qi – is like water. When it moves freely it stays clean and healthy. When it stops moving it becomes a breeding ground for all kinds of diseases. The Five Animal Frolics was part of the beginning of the science of Qigong and the foundation of many future Qigong practices.

Our modern world is very fast and stressful. We sit on chairs all day long and stare at computers. We constantly have to juggle the pressure of work and family. This pressure creates a lot of emotional and physical pain. Our breathing patterns reflect the famous fight or flight response when our body is under stress. It thinks that in order to survive, it needs to tighten the muscles and get ready to run. The ancient teachings of Qigong can help us address these patterns in our body. Qigong practice will help us see how our mind works and make us aware of the choices our body is making. It will train us to build positive patterns instead of negative ones. Qigong and Tai Chi are an investment and a gift for life.

Many people don't know that our bodies are built for a lot more physical activity than most of us get in our modern lives. We all know that exercise is good for our health and we all want to have a healthier life style. Some of us take up jogging, go to the gym a few times a week or take a kickboxing class. All of these exercises can be great for our heart and muscles but can lack emotional value, relaxation and a feeling of inner harmony. While we jog we usually listen to music and disconnect from our bodies. This type of exercise can also be painful and strenuous, even leading to joint damage as you age. When you do these kinds of exercises your body and mind are not in harmony. In order for us to evolve physically and emotionally we need a practice that answers both these aspects. The gentle effective movements of Qigong and Tai Chi can provide the solution.

This book serves as an introduction to the basic teachings of Qigong. You will learn the history of this ancient art, its philosophy, the main branches of Qigong and the movements. The book presents three main workouts: a short morning practice, the Eight Pieces of Brocade and finally, 18 Tai Chi Qigong form. These wonderfully simple exercises will quiet your mind, open up your spine and release tension in your joints and will help prevent injuries by bringing more awareness to your body. These workouts are ideal for people who don't have the time to spend days trying to learn the more complex poses of Tai Chi but still want to experience and feel meditation in motion for health.

These exercises can also serve as warm-up exercises for martial artists or anyone who is cross training. The goal of this book, as the title suggests, is to make you physically stronger and emotionally calm and balanced.

Chapter One

Brief History of China

In order to understand Qigong it is helpful to have some background on the history, cultural traditions and belief system of where it was born. China has one of the oldest civilizations in the world, with a recorded history of nearly 5,000 years. China is almost the same size as the United States, surpassed only by Russia and Canada. What seemed to keep China together and stable was its powerful bureaucracy. China developed her own culture from the beginning in her own way, with few decisive influences from abroad that were due to its geography.

Geography

Most of China is mountainous and hilly. All rivers flow into the Pacific Ocean, except the Huai River. There are five major rivers in China; the largest two are the Yellow River (named after its color) in North China and the Yangzi (which means large river, 3,964 miles) River in Central China. Generally, people consider the river a dividing line between North China and South China.

There are many differences between North and South China. The north has dry, cold, desert wind in winter. Horse riding was common. There farmers grow millet, barley, soybeans and wheat. The growing season is four to six months. The south has a moist climate with more plains, mountains and rivers. In the southern hills and valleys they grow rice, tea, mulberry trees for silkworm food and bamboo. The common way of transportation is by boat. There is common saying: "southern boats and northern horses." The southern season may last from nine months to a year. The northern famers tend to stay at home. Many men of the south are fishermen and traders and have traveled overseas. Hence, most Chinese in New York, London, etc., are mainly from the south.

The People

Seventy five percent of the Chinese population lives in the countryside, villages and small towns. The population of China consists of five groups: Han, Chinese; Man, Manchus; Meng, Mongolians; Hui, Muslims; and Zang, Tibetans. The Han, or pure Chinese, make up about 94% of the total population. Those in the north are taller by an average of two inches and have less yellow complexion. The principal regional differences, however, are marked by variations in dialect. The written language is held in common and can be read by all scholars. Chinese script first appeared about 1300 B.C.

Foundations of Chinese Civilization

The Chinese built a civilization that has lasted longer than any other in the world. In 5000 B.C., Chinese lived in the fertile Huang He river valley. In the 1700's B.C., invaders called the Shang entered their valley. These invaders built the first permanent, organized civilization. Since the Shang takeover, China has mostly been ruled by dynasties. The founder of the Ming dynasty brought China under one rule. Later, his grandson rebuilt the capital and renamed it Beijing. He also built a palace complex called the Forbidden City. The city got this name because only the rulers and a few officials could enter it. In 1664, the Manchus invaded China, creating the Qing dynasty. This lasted until 1911.

Achievements of the Dynasties

China has given the world some important inventions, such as paper, pottery called porcelain and silk cloth. The process of making silk was a very profitable industry. Caravans carried the precious cloth to Europe and Southwest Asia along a route called the Silk Road. Other traders carried porcelain, tea and spices. Travelers on the Silk Road faced danger from robbers, bad weather, lack of water and sickness. The Chinese developed a form of writing during the Shang Dynasty. The Great Wall and the Grand Canal were important feats of construction.

In China, slave society began around the 21st century B.C. Over the next 1,700 years, agriculture and animal husbandry developed greatly and the skills of silkworm-raising, raw-silk reeling and silk-weaving spread widely. Bronze smelting and casting skills reached a relatively high level and iron smelting became increasingly sophisticated. The Chinese culture flourished as a great number of thinkers and philosophers emerged, most famously Confucius. The written history of China begins with the Shang Dynasty (1600-1050 BCE). Two important events mark this period: development of a writing system, as revealed by inscriptions found on tortoise shells and oracle bones, and the use of bronze metallurgy. Each new dynasty claimed legitimacy by the possession of Mandate of Heaven.

In 221 B.C., Qin Shi Huang, the first emperor of the Qin Dynasty, established a centralized, unified, multi-national feudal state. This period of feudal society continued until after the Opium War in 1840. During these 2,000 years, China's economy and culture continued to develop, bequeathing a rich heritage of science and technology, literature and the arts. The four great inventions of ancient China - paper-making, printing, the compass and gunpowder - have proved an enormous contribution to world civilization.

Chinese civilization peaked during the Tang Dynasty (618-907) when Tang people traded with people all over the world. This is why Chinese residing overseas often call themselves Tang Ren, or the People of Tang.

In 1840, nervous to continue its opium trade in China, Britain started the Opium War against China. After the war, the big foreign powers forcibly occupied "concessions" and divided China into "spheres of influence"; thus, China was transformed into a semi-colonial society. The cultural climate was changing after 1900 and the failed Boxers' Rebellion, when the martial artists failed to remove the European and Japanese from Beijing. Modern technology seemed more powerful than the old ways.
In 1911, the middle-class democratic revolution led by Dr. Sun Yat-sen abolished the feudal monarchy and established the Republic of China, therefore starting the modern history of China.

In 1949 the Chinese Communist Party established the People's Republic of China, driving the Nationalist Party to Taiwan Island. In 1978 China adopted the Open Door policy, ending its long history of self seclusion.

Basic Elements of Traditional Chinese Beliefs

Buddhism, Daoism and Confucianism have been collectively called the "Three Doctrines" and together they have had a profound influence on Chinese culture and history. Buddhism came from India. Daoism and Confucianism are considered complementary traditions. Daoism is often thought to emphasize the yin aspects of reality and Confucianism the yang (powerful, order). Together they form a unity of opposites. They will be discussed separately. Daoism and Confucianism grew up together and actually, as they developed, helped generate each other. [1]

We first need to learn some of the features of traditional Chinese belief and practice. These elements provided a basis for later development of Chinese Medicine and are important to the development of Qigong and other Chinese Martial Arts.

Spirits – Early Chinese belief included the power of sprits. They believed the spirits are active in every aspect of nature.

Veneration of ancestors – The same respect that was given to spirits was given to the ancestors. At death, ancestors became spirits who needed to be placated to ensure their positive influence of living family members. Veneration of ancestors provided a soil for the growth of Confucianism.

Seeing pattern in nature – To survive, Chinese people had to learn that while they could not control nature, they could learn to work with it once they understood its patterns. Some patterns are easy to see: day and night, cycle of birth and death. Others are more subtle to see like the motion of waves, yin and yang.

---

[1] John Keay. *China: A History*, New York: Basic Books, 2011.

Chinese believed that a person has two souls, the *po*, "animal soul" or "life soul" and the *hun*, "spiritual/personality soul." Both souls become separated from the body at death and both of them can be kept alive by sacrifices upon which they feed. If the *po* is neglected, it may become a "demon" and hunt the living. Hence, the importance of having a male descendant to perform the family sacrifices.

***Yi Jing* (I Ching),** *The Book of Changes* (1122 BC).[2] It's an ancient book that interprets life through analysis of hexagrams. A hexagram is a figure of six horizontal lines. There are two kinds of lines: divided and undivided. Sixty four different hexagrams are possible and the *I Ching* gives an interpretation of each hexagram. A person can use the interpretation in making future decisions.

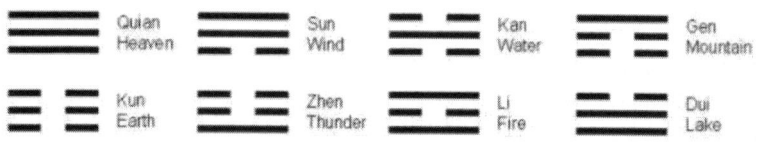

```
═══ Quian      ═ ═ Sun       ═ ═ Kan       ═══ Gen
═══ Heaven     ═══ Wind      ═══ Water     ═ ═ Mountain

═ ═ Kun        ═ ═ Zhen      ═ ═ Li        ═══ Dui
═ ═ Earth      ═══ Thunder   ═══ Fire      ═ ═ Lake
```

Figure 1: The Eight sacred Symbols, Gua.

The trigrams are related to the five elements of Wu Xing, used in **Traditional Chinese Medicine**. Those five elements are wood, fire, earth, metal and water.

Daoism vs. Chinese Folk Religion

Because it incorporated the basic elements of traditional Chinese beliefs and practices, Daoism is really like a shopping cart filled with a variety of items: observations of nature, philosophical insights, guidelines for living, exercises for health, etc. It should be noted that Daoism and Chinese folk religion are not exactly the same thing.

---

[2] Some historians date this book as far as 2400 BC.

Origins of Daoism

Unlike Confucianism, with its stress on human relations, Daoism is preoccupied with man's place in the natural world. In this form of Nature mysticism, the secret for man is simply to abandon self-effort and ease himself into the rhythm of the universe, the cycle of the seasons and the progression of day and night.

The origins of Daoism are not clear. Its earliest documents contain many points – healers, appreciation for hermit life, long life, breathing, meditation and trance.
Every movement needs a founder and Daoists trace themselves back to a legendary figure named **Laozi** (Lao Tzu), whose name means "old Master" or "Old Child." Whether Laozi ever existed is unknown. He may have been a real person or the combination of historical information about several figures or a mystic creation.

In the traditional story, Laozi's birth (600 BC) resulted from a virginal conception. He was born old – hence the name "old child." Laozi became a state archivist, keeper of the royal archives or a librarian, in the royal city of Loyang for many years. Eventually tiring of his job, Laozi left his post and traveled to the far west of China. At the western border, Laozi was recognized as an esteemed scholar and prohibited from crossing until he had written down his teaching.

The result was the *Daodejing* (Tao Te Ching), which can be translated as "The Classic of the Virtuous Way." The Daodejing is a short book of about five thousand Chinese characters. After Laozi was finished he left China and traveled westward. Stories told about his travels to India, later to return to China and his ascendency to the sky. He was soon treated as a God, the human incarnation of the Dao. He continues to be worshipped as divine by many Daoists.

Daoism and the Quest for Longevity

The challenge of facing our own mortality may very well be the ultimate test of being human. Next to the age-old questions relating to "the purpose of life" and the existence of God, coming to grips with the fact that we live this life and then, at some point, must die can truly stretch our intellectual limits.

The Daoists brought an interesting twist to immortality. They believed that it was truly possible to defy the entropic rules of nature and live beyond the standard program for life in this body. The old Daoist Masters believed that it was Qi (or Chi) that animated our physical bodies and kept us alive. This Qi existed throughout nature and to some degree, in all things. What we eat, drink, come in contact with and even "think" can affect the quality of our Qi.

These ancient teachers have known what modern science has only discovered in recent times, that our bodies and minds are fields of energy that move at different speeds and in different ways. These energy locations are interconnected and affect each other.

Various exercises that we now call **Qigong** (Chi Kung – life energy circulation) are the results of the work that these ancients developed to strengthen the body and spirit and help it to transcend the limits of the everyday. Some later forms of internal alchemy teach exercises that move the life force from its origin at the base of the spine upward toward the head. From there it circulates back, via the heart, to its origin. Today several popular physical disciplines continue this interest. Most influential is Tai Chi, a series of slow arm and leg motions thought to aid balance and circulation.

Chapter Two

Qigong Basics

"There is much more to the mind than just thinking. When your mind is silent, the universe surrenders."

Laozi

What is Qi?

In Chinese Qi (pronounced chee) means "life energy" or "life force," as well as "breath". Qi is a natural force that fills the world. Qi is in everything. Qi is the thing that gives life. In China it is an ordinary term and is a part of the common language. For example, if someone looks good, people will say he has strong Qi or the weather is called tien Qi (heaven Qi). Qi has been accepted in many cultures. In India it is called *Prana*; the Japanese call it *Ki* and the Native Americans, *the Great Spirit*. It's important not to think of Qi as being mystical, just to view it as internal energy. The energy in our body is real! The body is full of energy. When you focus your mind with some intention you will feel the difference. There are three main types of Qi according to the Chinese sages:

1. Heaven Qi (Tian Qi)
2. Earth Qi (Di Qi)
3. Human Qi (Ren Qi)

These were called San Cai (The Three Natural Powers). Energy from the Earth (Yang Energy) is drawn upward from the foot. Energy comes down from the Heaven (Yin Energy) through the crown of the head. Man is in the middle and needs to receive energy from both of these sources. A major concern of Daoists arts is connecting these two energies in order to utilize them for internal balance. In modern times we tend to forget that we humans are part of a larger cosmos. The focus of this book is about the history and the cultivation of the Human Qi.

All of these types of Qi interact with each other and influence one another. When Qi is balanced, the world is balanced and everything grows and prospers. When Qi is imbalanced there is negative energy and sickness. The world works in cycles and we need to adjust ourselves to work in harmony with these cycles to protect ourselves from harm and to lead healthier lives. This is the meaning of "Dao" which means "The Way." Knowing the way the world functions was always on the minds of Daoists and early Chinese thinkers. From this philosophy they created exercise and movements to bring the body's Qi into balance with nature.

Another example of creative harmony with nature is Feng Shui which means "wind water" and together the words represent harmony and balance. Feng Shui is the art of choosing the location of things to work in synchronization with the natural cycles of the universe. Feng Shui was initially used to identify places for families to live in and to determine the best burial sites for relatives. Later it was used to site palaces, government buildings and other public monuments. It was used to help people decorate their homes and offices. Even cities were designed and built according to Feng Shui principles.

What is Qigong?

It's difficult to give an accurate translation to Qigong because both parts have countless meanings. The word Gong (also spelled Kung) is a general term which means "work," "practice" or "skill," like Gongfu (Kung Fu). In China any skill that is acquired through learning or practice is called Gongfu. Thus the term "Qigong" means "breathing exercise," "energy work" or the study of Qi that takes a long time. In other words, Qigong is the practice of learning to control the movement of the Qi energy internally by using your mind. Unlike most Western exercises where the mind is completely disconnected, with Qigong the mind is involved in every movement, thus making it an internal exercise.[3] The Chinese character for Qi signifies vapor or mist rising off of rice.

---

[3] Qigong should not be seen as simply a breathing exercise. Qigong puts a lot of emphasis on breathing but this is not the main objective.

Qigong is considered a branch of Chinese Medicine along with acupuncture, massage, nutrition and herbs. All these branches are looking to adjust the Human Qi flow. Qigong is a preventative practice that focuses on trying to prevent an illness before its starts. There is a saying in China: "A good doctor prevents a disease rather than curing it."

The Chinese believe that aches and pains are the result of a blockage in vital energy or Qi. If the energy becomes blocked illness may result. Needles can be inserted into the skin at special points to remove the blockage, which is the basis of acupuncture.

This preventative practice is different from Western medicine which is built around the concept of people waiting to get sick, then going to see a doctor. Generally the more people get sick, the more money is made. Today in the West people are more dependent on pharmaceutical drugs to alleviate pain, lower anxiety, kill germs, etc. Every night we see many commercials that tell us about a new drug that will take our pain and aches away. We need to understand that drugs remove the pain only temporarily. Eastern medicine reminds us that healing can come from the inside. In order to heal we need to find the root cause of the problem and remove the pattern of the illness.

Qigong is a simple and practical approach to become skilled in matters of health, happiness and spiritual attainment. Qigong practitioners learn how to tap into their own inner resources and become self-sufficient and skilled at working with their own internal energy.

Qigong is based on the premise that the human body is an energy system. According to Chinese medicine all living things have Qi. As long as it has energy, or Qi, the body is alive. A healthy person has more Qi than an unhealthy person.

As a moving meditation, Qigong can be regarded as a mindfulness practice combining concentration and present-centered awareness. It is a way to prevent disease and improve health as a mindful approach to movement, help lower stress, increase energy, improve concentration, raise body awareness, promote relaxation and decrease the incidence of injury. Qigong exercises also strengthen the body: the bones, the organs, the muscles, blood circulation and the overall breathing process.

History of Qigong

The earliest beginnings of Qigong are unknown and steeped in mystery and legendary figures. It was a time when people depended on wind, water and animals for survival. The first type of this practice probably emerged naturally from people who worked the land. As we discussed earlier, the early Daoists and other Chinese philosophers were looking for patterns in nature and tried to work in harmony with the land. Some of the information about the cycles of nature has been written about in the *I Ching* (*Book of Changes*). It was probably the first book which talked about Qi in humans and nature, including basic ideas how to anticipate a season, when will it rain, etc. Qigong exercises were created to bring the body Qi in tune with nature and the seasons. It was also created from the quest for longevity, spiritual needs and a healthier life style.

The documented history of what we know as Qigong goes back approximately 2,400 years, but there are references archaeologists and historians to Qigong-like techniques which are 5,000 years old. The most commonly used early name for these practices was 'Dao-Yin', which can be interpreted as "leading and guiding the energy." It was also called Tu-Na which means adjustment for breathing and Neigong which means internal exercise. The name "Qigong" was not in general use until the 1950s.

Laozi discussed several breathing methods in the *Daodejing*. He claims that by concentrating on the Qi a practitioner will achieve suppleness and feel like a child.

The second most famous Daoist after Laozi was Zhuangzi ("Master Zhuang"), who lived around the 4th century B.C. during the Warring States Period (770-221 B.C.). Zhuangzi described the relation between a healthy lifestyle and good breath. He talked about breathing, to expel the old and ingest the new, mimicking animals, as a way to achieve longevity. He is also one of the first people to mention a Dao Yin practice.

Huang Ti (The Yellow Emperor) is considered the originator of many health practices linked to Qigong. His teachings were recorded in a text called *The Yellow Emperor's Classic of Internal Medicine*, which first appeared in writing about 300 B.C. and is still considered the most famous book on Chinese medicine.

From 200 B.C. to 500 A.D., Buddhism and yoga meditation techniques were brought into China and absorbed into the Chinese culture.[4] The Buddhist monks taught Qigong exercises, including still or passive meditation known as Chan (Zen). This marked a turning point in the Qigong world.

These techniques, along with Daoist internal alchemy teaching and Daoist philosophy, brought a new era to Qigong which began to be practiced at a deeper spiritual level. Historical documents tell us that Qigong-like practices were common in royal and noble households from ancient times. For hundreds of years, however, they were never taught to laymen. Only in the last hundred years have they been available to the general public.[5]

In 1973, archaeologists found one of the oldest drawings of Dao-Yin movements (168 B.C.). The drawing consists of 44 color illustrations of human figures performing therapeutic exercises, with accompanying captions. It has 44 human images, each 9-12 cm tall, arranged in four rows, with eleven images in each row. The drawing was named: *Dao Yin Tu* (the Dao Yin illustrations).
The image shows people doing stances, movements and self massage. They mainly show standing poses, but some show people bending forward, stretching and twisting. Some of the discernible words next to the figures in the drawing tell us how to move the body. Others have animal names next to them. With this finding it finally became possible not only to read about ancient Dao Yin but to actually see how it looked! And what's interesting is that most of the exercises in the drawing resemble modern Qigong movements.

---

[4] Yoga has much in common with Qigong and it might have influenced some of Qigong movements. Both Yoga and Qigong emphasize relaxation, breath, stretching and inner energy work.
[5] Ellae, Elinwood. *Qigong the Basics, (Tuttle Martial Arts Basics)*, Boston: Tuttle Publishing, 2004, P, 14-16.

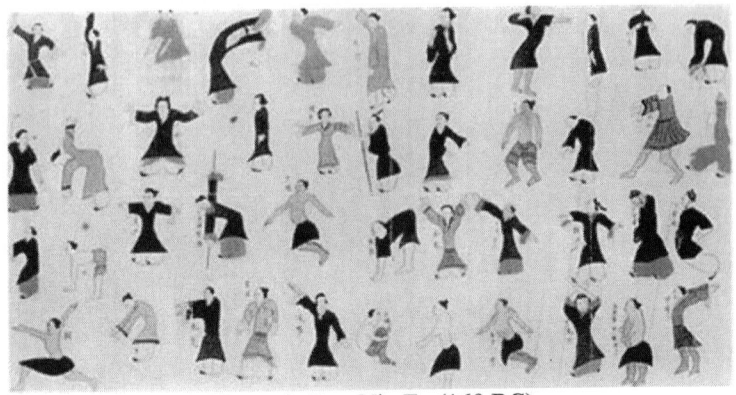

Figure 2: Dao Yin Tu (168 BC)

The famous physician Hua Tua (110-207A.D.) was known as the "Father of Chinese Medicine." He was the first in China to use acupuncture for an aesthesia during surgery. He also created the Wu Qin Xi (Five Animal Frolics), which is the oldest Qigong system still practiced today, dating back 2000 years. The idea behind the Five Animals is that people have become cut off from nature for a long time. Once they were isolated from nature they lost their animal instincts and the feeling of nature. Being removed from nature also means that humans don't know how to protect themselves or how to maintain their health. Animals on the other hand are connected to their bodies. They know how to move in the right way and how to survive in the wild. By imitating the movements of animals we can get our connection back and keep our bodies healthy. We can tune into the things we have forgotten.

The Five Animals are integral to the Five Elements Theory commonly used in acupuncture. The Bear emphasizes the spleen, the Tiger the liver, the Bird the lungs, the Ape the heart and The Deer the kidneys. In the Five Animals practice, we imitate the movement of each animal with special focus on its related organ system.

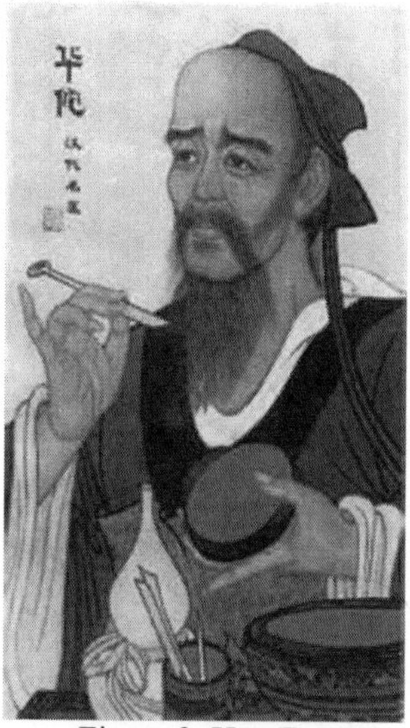

Figure 3: Hua Tua

One of the biggest influences in Chinese healing and martial arts came from an Indian Buddhist monk Da Mo (also known as Bodhidharma). Da Mo was born around 440 A.D. He was the third child of King Sugandha and was a member of the warrior caste.

In most of East Asia today, Da Mo is revered as the spiritual father of Zen Buddhism in China. He started what eventually became the Ch'an school of Buddhism in China (known as Zen in Japan and the West).

During the Chinese Southern Liang Dynasty (502-557 A.D.) the Emperor invited Da Mo to preach Buddhism in China. He eventually met Emperor Wu at Chin-ling (now Nanjing). After the Emperor decided he did not like Da Mo's Buddhist theory, Da Mo withdrew to a Shaolin Temple in Henan Province in northern China. Entering the temple he saw that the priests were in very poor health. Da Mo devised a series of exercises to strengthen and invigorate the monks. Some say he wrote two classics: I Chin Ching (Muscle/Tendon Changing Classic) and Hsi Sui Chin (Marrow Washing Classic). Da Mo's teachings instructed the Shaolin priests how to gain health and change their physical bodies from weak to strong (muscle/tendon changing), how to use Qi to strengthen the blood and immune system, and to energize the brain and attain enlightenment (marrow washing). The monks transformed from a group of physically weak men into a group of powerful and vibrant men. It's important to understand that in ancient times physical strength was a matter of survival not just health. The basis of these works, the physical drills of which are called Eighteen Hands of the Lohan (Buddha), were incorporated into the Shaolin Qigong and what became known as Shaolin Kung Fu martial arts.

During the Song dynasty (960-1279 A.D.) legend tells about Zhang, San-Feng as the person who created the most famous internal martial art: Tai Chi Quan. Apparently, the inspiration for Tai Chi came to him when he watched a fight between a crane and a snake. Although there is evidence that Zhang did exist, there is no evidence to support the theory that he was the creator of Tai Chi as we know it today. Exercises similar to Tai Chi and Qigong have existed in China for thousands of years. Most evidence points only to Tai Chi having been created only around the early 17th century by General Chen Wanting (1580-1660) the leader of the Chen family.[6] Chen Tai Chi is characterized by slow flowing movements (yin), followed by fast explosive movements (yang).

In the 11th century Dr. Wang, Wei-Yi[7], was the first to organize acupuncture theory and principles. Before that time acupuncture theory was very confused and unclear. Dr. Wang provided a clear illustration and explanation of the 12 Qi meridians (energy pathways) in the body. Dr. Wang explained the relationship of the 12 organs and the 12 Qi channels, clarified many of the points of confusion and for the first time systematically organized acupuncture theory and principles. In 1034 Dr. Wang used acupuncture to cure the emperor and with the support of the emperor, acupuncture flourished. Dr. Wang contributed to the advancement of Medical Qigong and Qi circulation theory.

---

[6] Mark Chen. *Old Frame Chen Family*, Berkley: Blue Snake Books, 2004. P, 9-12.
[7] Chinese names begin with the family name. Therefore Wang, Wei-Yi, would be called Wei-Yi Wang in the West because Wang is his last name.

The Eight Pieces of Brocade (Ba Duan Jin), also called the Eight Treasures or the Eight Silken movements, is one of the oldest and most classical Qigong forms created around $11^{th} - 12^{th}$ century. From then until the end of the Qing Dynasty, many other Qigong styles were founded.

During the Qing Dynasty (1644-1912) Tibetan meditation and martial techniques became widespread in China for the first time.[8] The third major internal martial art style to develop in China after Tai Chi and Xing Yi was Bagua Zhang (Eight Trigrams Palm) and includes elusive, swift changes of posture and direction. Bagua is believed to have been created by Dong Hai-Chuan (1813-1882). Bagua was designed to fight up to eight opponents at once. It is also known for its distinctive Qigong training method known as "walking the circle."

The concealment around Qigong teachings led to thousands of different styles. Each family or village, each religious or martial-arts group, in different areas of the country, developed their practices separately and passed them down only to a selective group within their own family or students. A few examples of distinct styles are Chen Tai Chi, Yang Tai Chi, Five Animal Frolics, Eight Pieces of Brocade and Bone Marrow Cleansing.

Modern Qigong

Modern Qigong was born after the Communist Revolution in 1949. During the Revolution, China lost half of its medical personnel (Western and Traditional). The Communist leaders lacked resources and money after a long war. They could not provide basic medical treatment to sick soldiers. A regional party leader heard how Liu Guizhen, a young party member, was cured of several illnesses by a local healer. Guizhen reported the healing powers of Neiyang-gong (inner cultivation). He also became a student and later a sixth-generation Master of the Neiyang-gong tradition. The Communist leaders were particularly pleased that the new techniques were simple and inexpensive.

---

[8] Jonathan Bluestein. *Research of Martial Arts*, Create Space Independent Publishing Platform, 2014.

On March 3, 1949, "Qigong" was proclaimed as the official name for the health exercises that Liu Guizhen and the group had developed.[9] Liu Guizhen is sometimes called "The Father of Modern Medical Qigong." In September 1957, Liu Guizhen's Qigong Therapy Practice was published. Thus Qigong practice began to spread among party members who then started forcing top Tai Chi Masters to devise Tai Chi and Qigong programs for the health of the general public. This led to a creation of a national Tai Chi/Qigong program.

By the 1970s it was popularized as daily morning exercise practiced by thousands in parks all across China. Qigong was introduced to the West in 1973, when President Richard Nixon (to the surprise of the world) visited China and opened Chinese teachings to the rest of the world. By the 1980s it was one of the most popular sports in China. It's estimated that around 100 million people were participating in some form of it! China experienced what became known as 'Qigong fever.' (Qigong re).[10]

One of the most famous movements to emerge during this period was the Falungong movement (even though its practice is not actually Qigong). Its leader, Li Hongzhi claimed that Qigong practice is not enough for those who want to achieve a higher level of fulfillment. There is a need for a moral strictness and the Law of the Dharma Wheel Practice (Falungong). He began to teach that the purpose of physical practice was not for good health, but spiritual salvation. The movement grew to millions of followers.
In 1999 a small magazine published an article criticizing the Falungong practice. In response 6,000 protestors stormed the magazine which then led to a mass demonstration by other Falungong members. At this stage the government saw the movement as a direct threat on the state and from that point the members of the group have been persecuted by the government. In

---

[9] For thousands of years the term "Qigong" has not been used to describe the energy practices of breath and movement which today is called "Qigong." Many other terms were used instead, most notably Daoyin meaning leading and guiding.
[10] David Palmer. *Qigong Fever*. New York: Columbia University Press, 2007. P, 154.

October 1999 the government declared Falungong a "heretical organization." Hundreds of thousands of members were sent to jail or faced harsh punishment. Li Hongzhi moved to the United States and the movement still has millions of followers around the world.

After the Falungong incident, the Chinese government took control of Qigong practice. Only state certified instructors were allowed to teach it. They also allowed only classical medical Qigong exercises such as the Eight Pieces of Brocade, Five Animal Frolic, etc. Many Qigong teachers moved to the West which helped spread Qigong in the West. In addition, the yoga-explosion over the last few decades has made America more open to the idea of mind-body exercises in general. Many people find similarities between the practices.

As for China, after the Qigong fever was over many of its citizens went back to the parks and practiced state sponsored exercises such as Tai Chi, dancing, senior couple dancing, etc. Qigong and Tai Chi are the only mind body or internal energy systems to be practiced and have worked for millions of people in the country where the system was invented. In India, by contrast, Yoga is practiced only by less than one percent of the population.

Qigong Theory

This section will discuss the basic theory and principles of Qigong practice. The basic theory will give us a better understanding of our practice. The Qi in our body cannot be seen but it can be felt. Imagine a car that runs on a battery. Our body is the car and the Qi is the battery. Without the battery the car does not work. It's the same with Qi in our body.

How does Qi move in our body? According to Chinese Medicine the human body has twelve major channels, called "meridians," and eight vessels through which the Qi moves. The twelve meridians – three Yin meridians of the hand, three Yin meridians of the foot, three Yang meridians of the hand and three Yang meridians of the foot.

The twelve major channels are like waterways which the Qi flows through our bodies. Six of them are connected to the fingers and the others are connected to the toes. The meridians transport vital energy to every cell, internal organ and muscle in the body. When the Qi in channels are full, the flow of Qi in the waterways is strong. When the Qi flow is slow or stagnates in the twelve rivers, the body is not balanced and this might lead to sickness.

When a person is sick, according to Chinese Medicine their Qi level is too aggressive (Yang) or too passive (Yin). A Chinese general practitioner will use acupuncture or herbs to bring the body back into balance between yin and yang. Another way of solving the problem is doing Qigong exercise which some doctors prescribe to their patients. Qigong can be used as preventative care to maintain health or to cure an existing health issue or injury.

According to Qigong theory a person is born with a certain amount of health capital or energy funds. Getting older, prolonged stress, major illness and injuries deplete one's life capital. Many of the changes that happen to us as we age are an indication of what's happening around us. In order to reverse the process or slow it down we need to get back to the source. Qigong can help make up this lost energy and also help people who are suffering from stress and depression.

Dao, Wuji and Tai Chi

According to Daoist philosophy the Dao is the original creative force of the universe. First there was stillness known as Wuji, – literally wu means 'no' and ji means "extreme." In western terms this could be compared to the time before the "Big Bang." In Daoist teachings there can be no stillness without movement, or the other way around, so eventually this stillness gave birth to the form of movement which is called Tai Chi. Tai Chi means 'grand extreme," which is the opposite of Wuji. As a famous Tai Chi saying goes "Wuji is the mother of Tai Chi." Tai Chi was born in the center of Wuji and started to spiral, thus Yin and Yang were born.

Yin and Yang

After about 1000 B.C. the Chinese commonly thought that the universe expressed itself in opposite but complementary principles:

day and night, hot and cold, sky and earth, male and female, left and right, etc. These complementary principles are Yin and Yang. Yin and Yang can be thought of as complementary (rather than opposing) forces that interact to form a dynamic system in which the whole is greater than the assembled parts. Everything has both Yin and Yang aspects. Another way to understand Yin and Yang is extremes of stillness and movement.

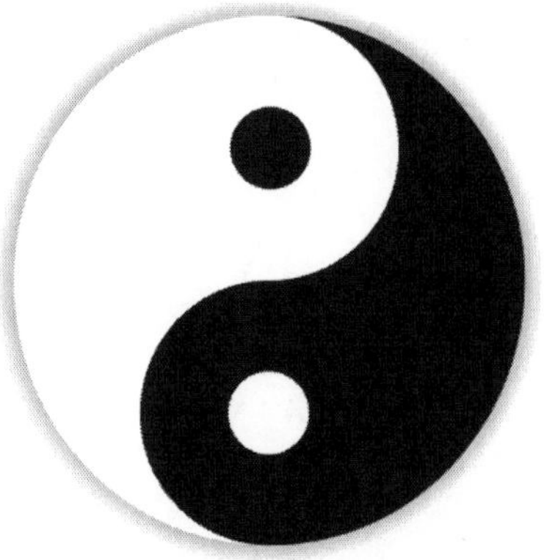

Figure 4: Yin and Yang Symbol

Yin is characterized as slow, soft, yielding, diffusive, cold, wet and passive. It is associated with water, earth, the moon, femininity and nighttime.

Yang, by contrast, is fast, hard, solid, focused, hot, dry and aggressive. It is associated with fire, sky, the sun, masculinity and daytime. Yang is the white part of the symbol, light like the sun. Yin is the black part, dark like the moon. Life naturally is not just made of extremes. When the spiraling energy of Tai Chi joins Yin and Yang what we get is the famous Tai Chi symbol in Figure 4.

Yin and Yang apply to the human body. In traditional Chinese medicine good health is directly related to the balance between Yin and Yang qualities within oneself. If Yin and Yang become unbalanced one of the qualities is considered deficient or has vacuity.

The Five Elements (The Wu Xing)

The interaction between Yin and Yang follows a natural cycle. The cycle operates with the Five Elements of nature – Water, Wood, Fire, Earth and Metal. Taken figuratively, these elements are the foundation of the material world. Taken symbolically, each one the Five Elements represents a movement of energy and they combine into a cycle of generation as shown in Figure 5. The cycle shows how each energetic movement creates a new energetic movement. Therefore, wood makes fire, fire creates earth, earth produces metal, metal nourishes water, and water makes wood. If, however, one element becomes too strong, an imbalance of Yin and Yang will happen. This will lead to blocked Qi. One way to prevent that is a Qigong workout.

Chinese Medicine regards the heart, liver, spleen, lungs and kidneys as the five internal organs, which line up with the five elements theory as shown in Figure 5. Similarly, a chronic emotional condition may have a physical impact on the organs. The Liver connects to depression and anger. The Heart connects to excess of joy. The Spleen connects to obsession. The Lungs connect to grief and suffering and finally, the Kidneys connect to a sense of fear.

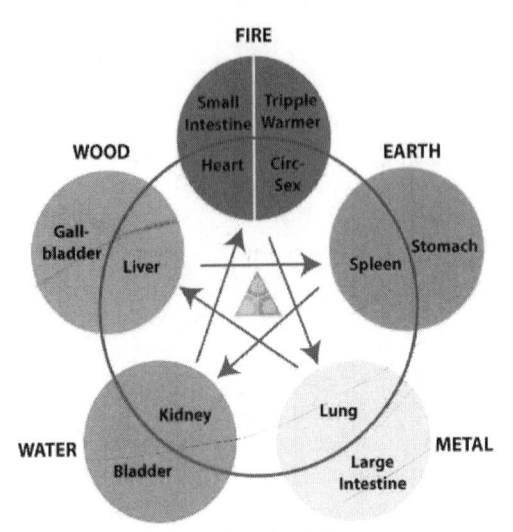

Figure 5: The Five Elements

To summarize, the Wu Xing can be seen as five movements which can take place in both the physical and the energetic sphere.

Dantian

According to Qigong theory, Dantian is the point in your body that is the center of gravity, breathing and energy. It is located between your pubic bone and your navel in the center of your abdomen. It is the store house of your body's energy, as well as the force that gets the energy moving to the specific places in your body where you need it.[11] The Dantian is not on the surface of the skin. You may compare it to a small ball located inside the lower abdomen. There are three Dantian points according to Qigong theory. Each one of them is associated with basic human functions:

1. Lower Dantian: located in the lower abdomen (about three inches below and two inches behind the navel) and stores sexual energy and vitality (Jing). When your lower Dantian is healthy and strong, your immune system is strong.

2. Middle Dantian: located in the center of the body around the heart and connects to the health of the internal organs and the spirit (Shen). When your middle Dantian is strong you become more loving to yourself and other people.

3. Upper Dantian: located on the forehead between the eyebrows and connected to the brain. It is associated with your power to think clearly. In Hinduism it is referred to as the third eye. When the upper Dantian is strong you have clear intuition and sharp vision.

The lower Dantian is the most important and is the most talked about of the three. If someone refers to Dantian without specifying the location they probably mean the lower Dantian.

For most people the three Dantians are imbalanced. Some people have powerful upper Dantian but weak middle Dantian. While

---

[11] Stanley Wilson. *Qigong for Beginners*, New York: Sterling Publishing, 1997. P. 29-30.

some people have a strong middle Dantian but have a weak lower Dantian. The question is how to balance all three. Is it possible to balance vitality, love and wisdom? The answer is yes, the Central Meridian runs through all three Dantians and connects your body with Heaven Qi and Earth Qi. Together the Central Meridian and the three Dantians are called the Golden Wheels. With all four running smoothly, your body functions in harmony and balance.

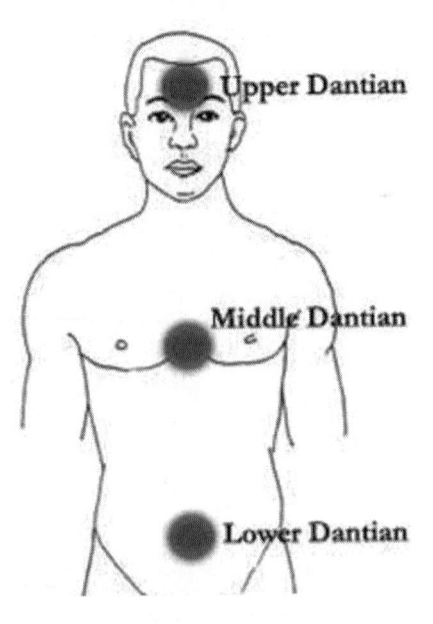

Figure 6: Three Dantians

Different Forms of Qigong

There are thousands of Qigong forms practiced around the world. Most are designed to promote health, but some focus on developing skill in martial arts. To keep things simple, Qigong can be divided into three main categories:

1. **Medical Qigong** (Yi Jia Gong), which is done to boost the immune system, health and for relaxation. As we mentioned earlier Qigong practice is meant to prevent an illness before it starts. Hua Tua claimed that the doctor's job was to keep the patient healthy.

The patient's job was to take care of his own health, using the doctor as an advisor. Unlike western medicine, which diagnoses the disease once it has taken place, Chinese medicine combines doctors' advice with patients who are connected to their own health. Medical Qigong is the most popular form of Qigong and is the main subject of this book.

2. Spiritual Qigong (Jing Gong) also called Meditative Qigong, is done to enhance spiritual growth and achieve enlightenment. The focus is on trying to develop a clear mind and a deeper self awareness.

3. Martial Qigong (Wu Gong) in China is referred to as Wu Shu, which means martial arts. Martial Qigong is done to improve the student's strength, focus and fighting skills.

Qigong Training Principles

Hua Tua (110-207 A.D.) known as "the Father of Chinese Medicine," told one of his students, "The body should be exercised but not to excess." Exercise improves the digestion and keeps the meridians clear of obstructions. In this way, the body remains free of illness. A door hinge does not rust if it is frequently used.

A Qigong workout is a series of active postures or forms that flow fluidly from one movement to the next movement. The exercise also can include standing meditation, self massage, breathing practices, stretches and sitting positions. Whatever type of Qigong you are doing, there are important basic elements: correcting your posture, regulating your breath and calming your mind.

1. Correcting Your Posture

First you need to adjust your posture until it's relaxed, comfortable and balanced. A key point in good posture is to sink down the body. In Qigong as well as Tai Chi every part of the body seeks its lowest level. The hips sink, the shoulders sink, the abdomen sinks, the elbows sink and even the breath sinks down to the lower Dantian. Correct posture should include the following principles:

1. The top of the head should be suspended (as if a string is lifting the top of your head), the eyes should look forward and the chin slightly tucked in. The tongue should rest on the roof of the mouth. The whole body should be relaxed and loose.

2. Relax your waist and let it sink down naturally. The "Spinal Twist" exercise in the morning workout will help you loosen the waist.

3. The chest muscles should be relaxed, neither concave nor curved out.

4. Straighten the lower back. Tuck the pelvis in, meaning you need to move it forward.

5. Sink the shoulders and elbows, without forcing them. This will help you sink the body down and relax.

6. Knees should be slightly bent, with the total body relaxed, straight, and centered.

If you don't stand correctly, you create tension in your body. Maintaining good posture allows your mind to relax and creates a good Qi flow. As Bruce Lee wrote, "Proper posture is a matter of effective interior organization of the body which can be achieved only by long and well disciplined practice."[12]

Good posture starts from the ground. When you practice Qigong or any martial art you need to be rooted to the floor, like a tree is rooted to the earth. If you are not rooted you lose your balance. Balance is a combination of relaxation, rooting and centering.

2. Regulating Your Breath

Regulating your breath means to slow down the breath until your breathing is soft, deep and long. Breathing is connected to emotions. Anger makes our breath constricted. If we feel stressed

---

[12] Bruce Lee. *Tao of Jeet Kune Do*. Santa Clarita: Ohara Publication, Inc, 1994. P, 29.

our breath is short and shallow to the point that it appears almost nonexistent. This does not mean that you inhale or exhale to the maximum which can hinder your oxygen supply. You should inhale and exhale to about 75%, so the lungs have room to operate. The rib cage and chest should barely move while you are breathing. Allow your breath to be full and move deep into your abdomen. Key words for good breathing: Calm (Jing), Long, Deep, Slow and Soft. Deep and calm breathing relaxes you and keeps your mind sharp. The breath is a bridge between the body and the mind. Oxygen could be described as the most essential food.

Always breathe through the nose. In Qigong there is a saying, "The nose is for breathing, the mouth is for eating." By breathing through the nose you naturally penetrate deeper into your body.

3. Calming the Mind

When our mind is calm our breath slows down; therefore, to keep our breath calm we need to calm our mind. Meditation (passive or active) or breathing exercises in the beginning of our practice can help us slow down and calm our mind and our emotions. According to Daoist teachings, the hardest thing to learn is to stop thinking. Being constantly in our head is not good for us. The same way the body needs a rest after a long day of work, the mind needs a rest, too.

It is especially true in modern society when we have so much stimulation around us. We always think about the past or the future. Being in the moment is the first step of calming our mind. It allows us to forget about what we did before our practice or need to do after it. The next step is to slow down our thinking process and enjoy the now moment. When you reach this moment (and that might take some practice) your mind will be calm and light.

As you prepare for a Qigong or Tai Chi workout, you should stand still for 30 seconds with the head suspended and shoulders dropped. This will give the mind a feeling of relaxation. During the practice you should ask yourself "Am I relaxed? Am I calm?"

Important Qi Energy Points

The points of accesses to our bodies are known as acupuncture points. Every holistic school has different points, names and locations for the acupuncture points. But they all serve the same idea, that these points are a gateway into our internal system. By focusing our awareness on some of these points during our practice, we can help to balance the Qi in the body.

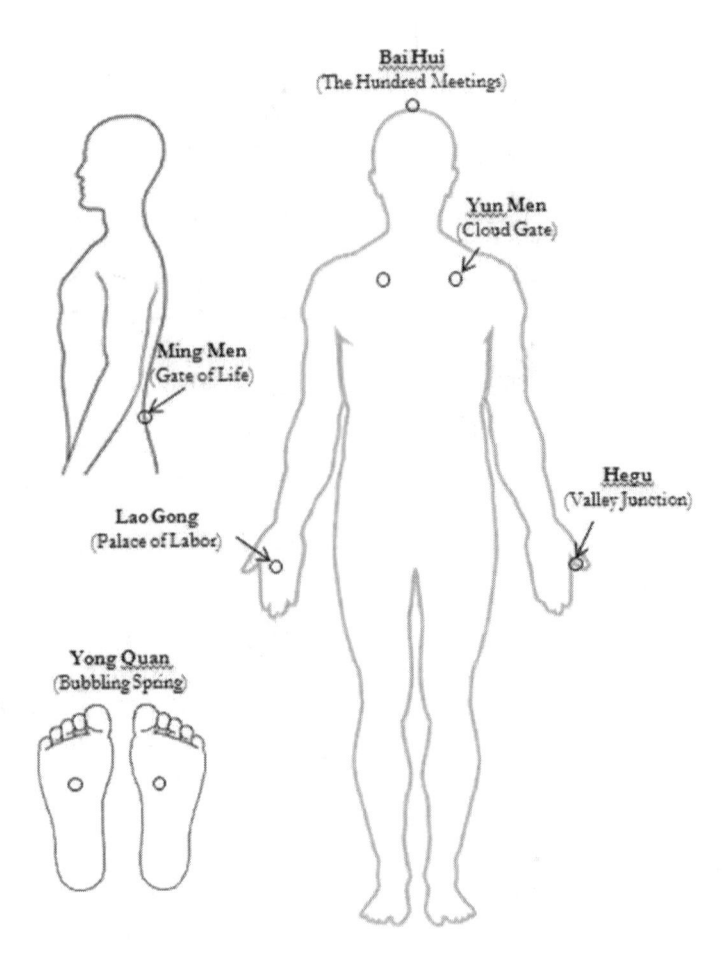

Figure 7: Qi Energy Points

Lao Gong (Palace of Labor or Work Palace)
Located in the center of the palms is a point for releasing energy and healing through the hands. Used to sense or send Qi, it's the easiest point to feel the flow of Qi.

Yun Men (Cloud Gate)
Points under the collar bone, which when massaged, bring relaxation.

Hegu (He, Junction; Gu, valley)
Points between the fourth finger and thumb bring relaxation to the body when massaged.

Bai Hui (Hundred Meetings or Hundred Channels)
Another point is located at the crown of the head. It's called the hundred meetings because many energy channels converge in the head. Sensing this point will help you position the head in the correct alignment with the body. Qi is directed to this point during meditation or some movements. In Yoga, this point is called the Crown Chakra.

Ming Men (Gate of Life)
The fourth point is on Governing Channel. It controls your kidneys and is located in your lower back opposite the navel. Focusing on this point is good for Qi stimulation and improves the kidney functions. You can also use your fists or hands to rub the area.

Yong Quan (Bubbling Spring or Bubbling Well)
This point is located in the center of the sole of the foot, just below the ball. Stimulating this point calms the spirit, promotes the Qi flow through the entire body and lowers blood pressure. You can massage the balls of the feet with your hands. This is good for relaxation and can help with insomnia. It's an acupuncture point on the meridian kidney.

Mind and Body Practice

Like Yoga, Qigong and Tai Chi are considered mind and body practices. In Traditional Chinese Medicine (TCM) there is a core belief that our health is merely a reflection of our state of mind. This is something that the Western Science is starting also to accept. When we feel stressed, we take shallow breaths and we find it hard to breathe. When we can't breathe, the symptoms of stress get worse and we feel more stressed. Negativity and tension affects our heart, brain, and our entire body. This will also lead your body to be stiffer. When your mind is relaxed, however, your body is relaxed. When we are relaxed and feel good, the breath becomes deeper, longer, and slower. Breathing is a process of absorbing a pure source of energy, oxygen, and eliminating the impure. Qigong will help you breathe better.

The words Emotion and Motivation are derived from the Latin root "to move." Think of the word emotion as standing for energy in motion! Both emotion and motivation literally move us and cause us to act. Emotions can be both physical and mental. Our practice and feelings are influenced by our emotion and state of mind during the practice. These days many people are repressed emotionally as they spend a lot of time learning to control their emotions. As time goes by we move further away from our natural state of being. How can we develop spiritually and emotionally if we forget who we are? Practicing Tai Chi and Qigong can help us connect and balance our emotion. Lack of movement leads to a lack of energy, stress leads to anxiety, depression, etc., but it's not just stress, it's how we deal with stress – sleeping too much, eating too much, shopping and staying on the computer for too long.

Historically, in nature, we had to survive in a hostile environment either from animals or the harsh weather. This is where we developed the fight or flight response to an attack or any threat to our survival.[13] However, in modern times it's not life threatening events that cause us to panic, but regular day to day activities such talking in public that get us into fight or flight mode. The problem is that our body doesn't know it! Over time this stress is very dangerous to our health. Moreover, the fight or flight response that our bodies developed a long time ago, was built for a short event, not long events. Today we find ourselves in long stressful situations like deadlines, job interviews, traffic jams, etc. These long periods of stress are very harmful to our immune system.

---

[13] Walter Bradford Cannon. *Bodily changes in pain, hunger, fear, and rage.* New York: *Appleton-Century-Crofts.* 1929.

Internal Exercises vs. External Exercises

Qigong, like Tai Chi, Xing Yi and Bagua, is an internal art or internal exercise. Internal exercises, active or passive, train you to feel the physical and energetic states of your body and how they influence your mind. Internal exercises build up and balance energy levels. In contrast, external exercises like running, karate, swimming, boxing, etc., are mainly aerobic and are meant to increase your heart rate and strengthen your muscles and keep you in shape. Internal arts teach you to use stillness of the mind for relaxation or to win a violent fight.[14] A major advantage of internal systems is that a blockage of Qi flow or blockage of stress can be opened up without force, which can be harmful to the body.

Yoga is also an internal exercise which uses postures (asanas) and breath-control (pranayama) to strengthen and energize the body. There are many similarities between the practices. In Hatha Yoga (classical Yoga), however, you stretch in order to relax the body and mind, while in Qigong you relax the mind in order to stretch.

The difference between Tai Chi and Qigong

Many people are confused about what the difference is between Tai Chi and Qigong. The short answer is Tai Chi is a Qigong, but Qigong is not Tai Chi. In other words, Tai Chi is a form of Qigong but its movements can also be used in full speed as a fighting art. Both systems are based on the principle of Chinese medicine and use the power of the mind and the cultivation of Qi. Tai Chi solo forms follow all of the guidelines for Qigong posture and Qigong breathing.

---

[14] Bruce Frantzis. *The Power of Internal Martial Arts and Chi: Combat and Energy Secrets of Ba Gua, Tai Chi and Hsing-I*, Berkeley: Blue Snake Books. 2007.

Chapter Three

Stances, Breath and Mind

Qigong Stances

The Qigong stance is the foundation for all Qigong exercises and also for standing meditation. The Qigong stance combines a light head, a lifted spine, deep breathing, feet rooted and training the mind to relax.

Standing Stances

In this book we will cover two basic stances that we will use in our Qigong practice. The first is the basic Qigong Stance, also known in Martial Arts such as Tai Chi, as Horse Stance. The second is Bow Stance, which is wider a stance.

1. Horse Stance (Ma Bu)

Starting with feet close together, connect to the ground through the feet. The hands are relaxed at the sides of the body and the head is lifted. Imagine your head is suspended by strings. As the classic expression goes "loosen the head and lift the crown of the head."

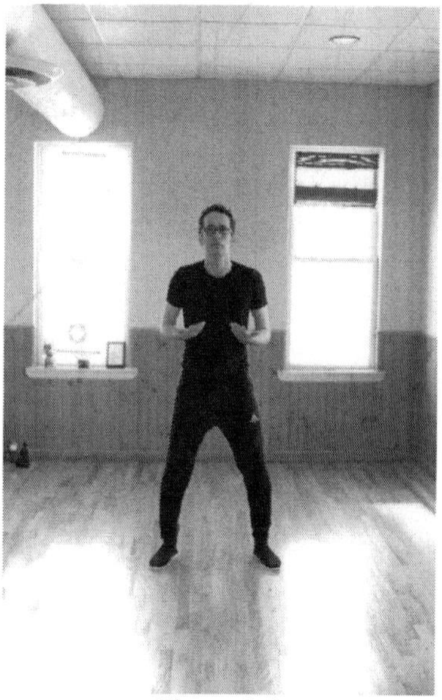

Figure 3.1

The chest is soft and relaxed, elbows relaxed, shoulders relaxed. The spine is long and open. Eyes are softly open. Abdomen is soft moving up and down with breath. The tongue is rested at the roof of the mouth.

Now to transition into horse stance, bend the knees, transfer the weight to the right foot, lift your left foot and step it to the left, coming down toes first and then lower the feet. You should be balanced between both feet and the feet should be parallel, meaning the distance between the toes is the same distance between the heels. Keep your chest, spine and shoulders loose.

Allow the breath to come in and out naturally. As a beginner you might not sink your knees too much. But as you progress in your practice, you will develop more leg strength and you will be able to sink the knees more.

2. Bow-Arrow Stance (Gong Jian Bu)

Bow stance is the most common stance in Tai Chi. Bring one leg forward. The knees and toes should be lined up perpendicularly. The rear leg is firmly down and a little bent, it should supporting 40 percent of the weight. Keep the upper body upright to the ground.

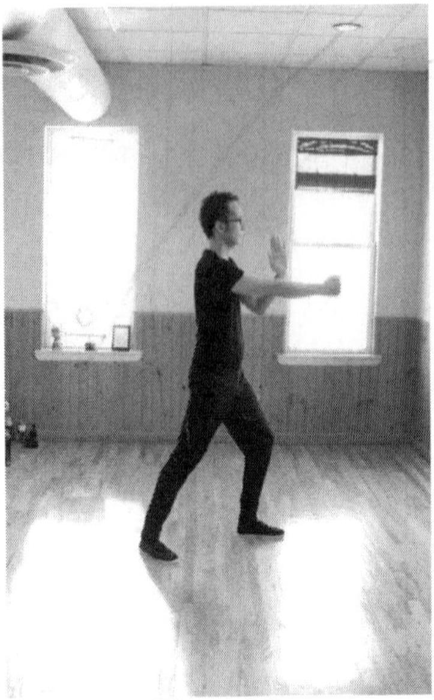

Figure 3.2

Meditation

Eastern teachings have brought two major breathing or mediating systems to the west.
1. Pranayama breathing (Yoga).
2. Daoist breathing (Qigong).

Both systems have several similarities such as seeking to extend the duration of the breath and having good posture while breathing. In pranayama, however, people are told to hold their breath. In Qigong breathing you never hold the breath. There are many forms of Daoist meditation. One of the most popular is the Wuji meditation.

Wuji is a form of deep meditation which can be done by sitting, standing or lying down. Like many other meditations it leads you to stillness, mental and physical relaxation. Many people can't see the value of sitting down in silence. Even though it seems inconsequential and unimportant, meditation can bring about many amazing results, such as: calming the mind, calming the body, enhancing focus, enhancing creativity, easing tension, etc.

Meditation is a practice of unwinding and coming back to a place of stillness and balance. Your goal is to find good breathing habits in all situations you may find yourself. When it comes to relaxation, there are two ways to achieve it:

1. Active Relaxation – also known as guided meditation. In Chinese it's called *cun si*: healing visualization. Here your brain is active and visualizes images and places. Some call it a "focused relaxation."

2. Passive Relaxation – here you are trying to empty your mind. In Chinese it's called *ru jing*: entering tranquility. This might be more challenging to some people and will take some time to get used to.

Meditation can be a challenge in the modern world. We are so stimulated with information which makes it hard sometime to clear our mind and to destress after a long day at work. According to eastern teachings, the cause of stress is not what happens to you, but how your mind responds to what happens to you. Sometimes the easiest way to relax is just to breathe.

Try to meditate before your morning practice, when you get back from work or before you go to sleep, provided that you are not too tired. If you meditate during these times then it's easier to keep the concern of the day out of your head.

Try to sit for a few minutes and concentrate on your breath and try breathing deeply. Deep breathing energizes the body, clears stress, calms the mind, increases lung capacity and deepens the meditation. Pay attention to your breath and to any internal sensations.
The rhythm of the breath should feel like a wave in the ocean going up and down. This how we should breathe, imitating the movement of the tide. Here are some guidelines and tips for a peaceful meditation:

1. Find a quiet and peaceful place where you will not be disturbed. Turn off all the electronics (cell phones, iPad, etc).

2. If you need some sound, you can play some quiet meditation music.

3. Sit whatever way is comfortable for you. Everyone thinks meditation is done by sitting with crossed legs. Not true - you can sit on chair, on a block on the floor or on a pillow.

4. Lift through the top of your head and drop your shoulders down. Imagine as if a string were lifting you by the top of your head. Try to maintain a straight and tall spine.

5. Put one hand on your belly and one hand on your chest. As you inhale and exhale move only your belly. Feel your lower abdomen expand. Most people breathe using their upper chest. Abdominal breathing is a key in Qigong and meditation practices.

6. Put the tip of your tongue to the roof of your mouth. Now take a slow deep breath through the nose. Follow the movement of air as it moves from your nose to your lungs and into your abdomen.

7. Do not hold your breath. Breathe softly in a relaxed way.

8. Visualize a relaxing and calming place such as a river or a forest and slow down your breath.

9. Try to make each inhale and exhale about the same length. Your breathing will begin to slow down.

Embrace the Tree (Standing Qigong)

Embrace the Tree is one of the most important and commonly practiced standing meditations in Tai Chi, Neigong and Qigong classes. Standing Qigong also known as Zhan Zhuang (standing post), is a method of developing internal strength and improving your health.

As Master Ken Cohen observed, "Standing Meditation is 'a million dollar secret.' It is a secret because it is so obvious, so ordinary that we do not give it any attention it deserves. It is hidden as the air is hidden."[15] In old times, a student could spend up to three years perfecting just Embrace the Tree.

This powerful technique increases internal awareness and opens the energy gates of the body and thus allows more Qi flow. The Chinese term for standing meditation is "Standing Post." It's also called the "three – circle posture," i.e., the arms, hands and legs are all bent to shape a circular posture. A feeling of vibration in the body is a sign of good posture.

1. Stand in horse stance. Shoulders are lowered and arms are relaxed, knees a little bent. The head is suspended as if it's pulled by a string. Find the center (meaning find the middle between back and forward).

---

[15] Kenneth S. Cohen. *The Way of Qigong*. Toronto: Ballantine, 1997. P, 134.

2. Then float your hands and elbows up to the level of your heart – elbows lower than wrists, palms facing your torso, creating a circle with your arms. Imagine you are hugging a big tree. Keep the hands and fingers apart. Try to focus on your lower Dantian. Look at a point directly ahead with relaxed eyes.

3. Breathe through the nose, taking the time to notice how each breath has a distinct quality of feeling. You may close your eyes. With a relaxed mind, notice any place you feel tight or achy (this could be blocked Qi). Try visualizing positive Qi moving to the area of discomfort and releasing the tension away. Try not to fidget.

4. Maintain this position anywhere between two to five minutes. Then work your way up to 15 minutes at a time. The mind should be peaceful and meditative. This form should not hurt your knees or lower back if done correctly. If there is stress on the knees, recheck your posture and adjust with calm.

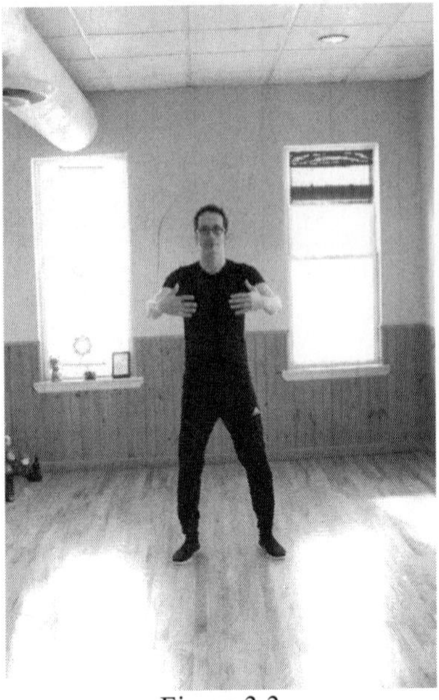

Figure 3.3

Advanced Standing Qigong

This is the more advanced standing meditation because it takes the most endurance to hold your arms up for a few minutes.

1. Stand in horse stance, shoulders relaxed, knees a little bent and unlocked. Keep the head upright, eyes looking forward, somewhat downward.

2. Lift your elbows just about shoulder level and bring the palm in front of your face. Relax your abdomen and breathe into your lower Dantian slowly and deeply.

3. Hold anywhere between one to five minutes.

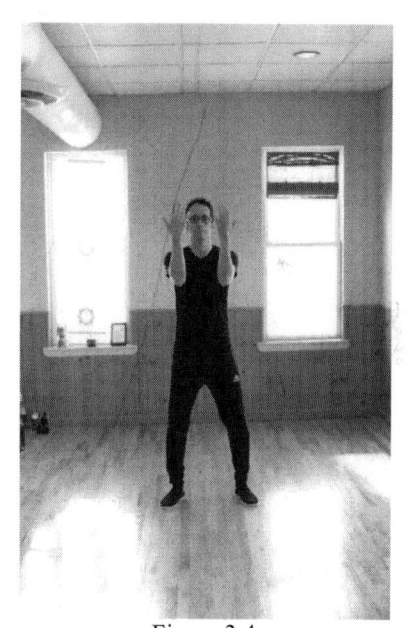

Figure 3.4

Once you meditate for a few minutes you will start to become aware of any stiffness or tension in your body, and you will be able to use the breath to release it. The key to a successful meditation session is not to force it and understand that it will take a while for you to experience all the wonderful benefits of peaceful breathing.

Lying Down Qigong

Lying down meditation is great for beginners, for people who suffer from insomnia, for people with back pains and relaxation at the end of you practice. It's also an effective way of learning how to breathe deeply.

1. Lie down on your back so that your spine is in a straight line. Your legs should be almost fully extended. The full length of the back should be flat on the floor.

2. Place one hand on your lower abdomen and one hand on your chest. On each inhale, breathe deep into the lower abdomen first, then into ribs, and then all the way up into the chest.

3. Exhale from top to bottom, releasing the air from your chest, then the ribs and finally the abdomen. At the bottom of the exhale, actively squeeze all of the air out. Breathe slowly and smoothly.

4. Concentrate your attention fully on the muscular movement. Continue breathing this way for 2 minutes.

Chapter Four

Morning Qigong

When to Practice

You can pick any of the three workouts in the book as they can be done any time of the day. The optimum time, however, to practice Qigong or Tai Chi is the early morning and on an empty stomach, anytime between 6:00am to 10:00am. The Qi is at its highest level, the body is relaxed and it will have more energy for the rest of the day. I like to practice in the morning after a cup of tea. If these times don't fit with your schedule, practice whenever it works for you. Early evening or when you get back from work is also a good time, but try to avoid exercising before going to bed.

The three workouts in this book can take anywhere between 5 and 15 minutes. The important thing is to practice each day. This will be easier if you set a certain time and a place for practice. The morning exercise is especially great for people with stressful jobs. If you work in an office try to spend 3-5 minutes doing spinal cord breathing, neck stretches and low back stretches during your break.

Warm Up

Like any workout, warming up is always a good idea. Because most of the movements presented in this book are low impact, a long warm up is not needed. Just one to three minutes should do it. These simple exercises are designed to loosen the main joints of the body. These exercises will also free up tension, and open blocked energy pathways of the body. A few options for a quick Qigong warm up include:

1. Self Massage (*An Mo Gong*) – Rub your hands together and between your fingers to generate heat and massage any areas of tension or pain.

2. Gently pat with your palms open (Lao Gong) or make loose fists with your hands and tap over all your body. Like a massage, the patting stimulates circulation and

releases stagnation in the body. Over time you can tap harder as your body gets comfortable with the tapping.

This tapping will open all the Qi channels in your body. Pat yourself up and down your front a couple of times. Tap the outside, and then down inside each arm three times. Starting right above the chest, tap down to hip area and back up again. Pat up and down the inside and outside of your legs. Bend over and tap both sides of the kidney area (lower back area). Tap these with your hands fully opened, trying to cover as much as you can with your hands.

3. Gentle stretching is also a great warm up. Standing up straight with your feet slightly more than hip distance apart, turn your shoulders and torso from side to side, letting your arms hang freely. Bend forward, hang and try to touch your ankles or your toes (Figure 4.1). Let gravity open and stretch your body. Relax your face and breathe. Slowly return to the standing position.

Make sure not to overstretch – go only as far as you feel comfortable even if you are unable to touch your toes.

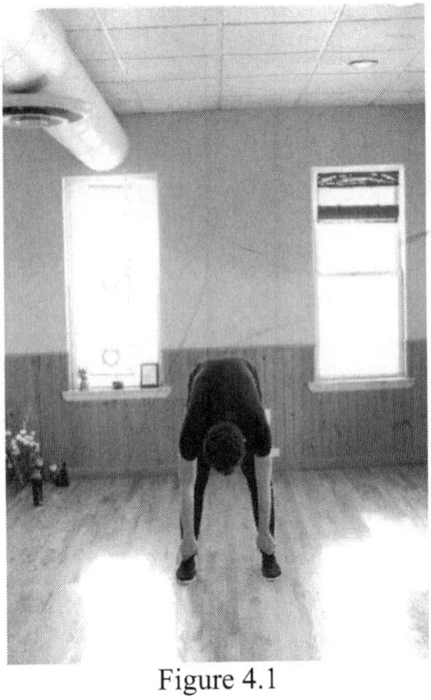

Figure 4.1

4. Frog Stance

Frog Stance, also known as squatting, helps lengthen the muscles of the lower back. It also increases ankle flexibility. Squatting used to be a very popular stance in ancient times but is seldom used today in the West. If you can't do a full squat, bend down as far as you can.

Stand with your feet shoulder-width apart. Bend your knees and lower yourself down into a squat. Next pull your elbows right under your knees. You can either bring your hands in prayer pose (Figure 4.2) or open the palms outwards (Figure 4.3). Hold the squat for 2 minutes.

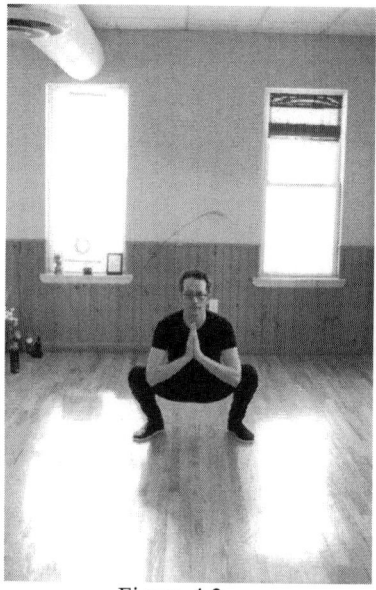

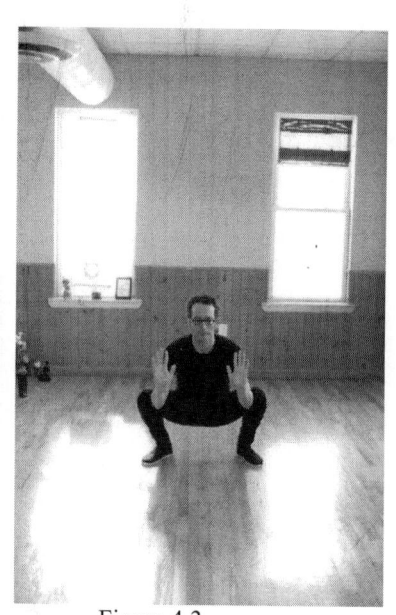

Figure 4.2   Figure 4.3

Morning Workout

Spinal Cord Breathing

This exercise is great for shoulder and neck pain. This movement is great for people who work in offices and sit most of the day.

1. Stand with legs shoulder-width apart. Clench the fists and bring your hands up in front of your face. Inhale and arch your back and look up.(Figure 4.3)

2. Exhale and round your back and tuck your lower back (Figure 4.4).

3. Inhale, open your arms, open your chest and look up.

4. Repeat 7-8 times. This exercise is good to open the tension in the lower back.

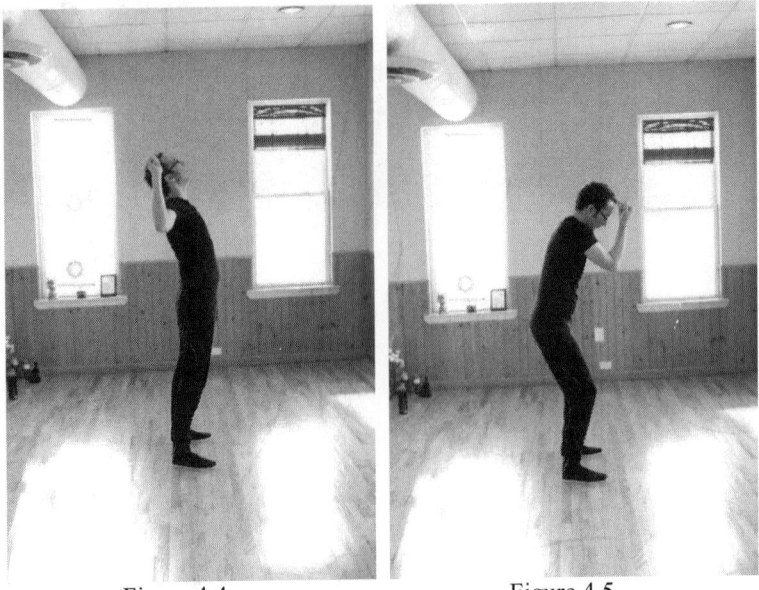

Figure 4.4   Figure 4.5

Lifting the Sky

This exercise is very good for the lungs and breathing as well as for back pains.

1. Stand with legs shoulder-width apart and bring your hands in front of your lower Dantian (2 inches below the navel), palms facing up.

2. As you inhale deeply, move your hands all the way over your head, keeping the elbows soft and the palms facing the ceiling.

3. On the exhale, float your hands back down to the starting position. Continue for 2 minutes.

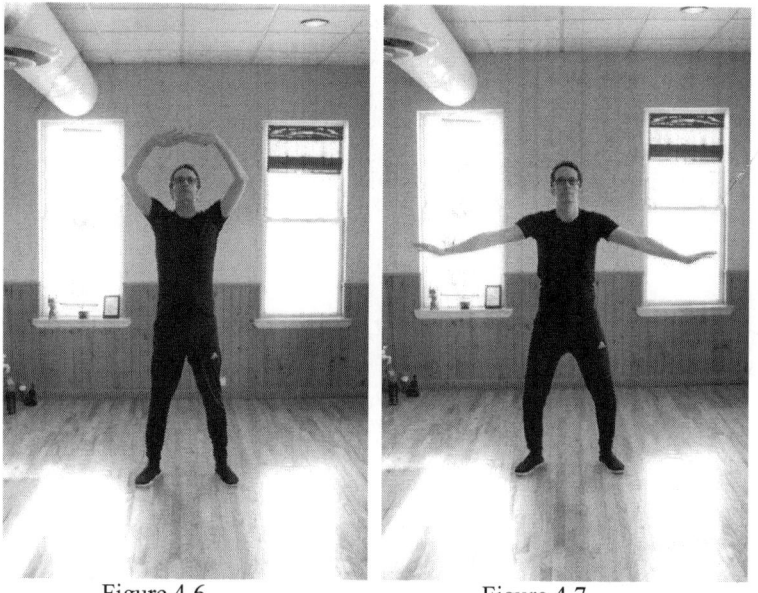

Figure 4.6   Figure 4.7

Neck Stretches

This exercise is great to release tension in the neck and the shoulders. It should be practiced very slowly. The neck is a crucial area, as many meridians pass through it.

1. Push your palms together behind your back with your fingers pointing down (reverse prayer pose). Begin slowly by lowering your chin into your chest. Next slowly move your left ear toward your left shoulder, then bring your chin toward your chest, and then bring your right ear toward your right shoulder.

2. Move the head back through the vertical position to start again. Move the head slowly, remembering to breathe throughout the exercise. Repeat 7-8 times in each direction.

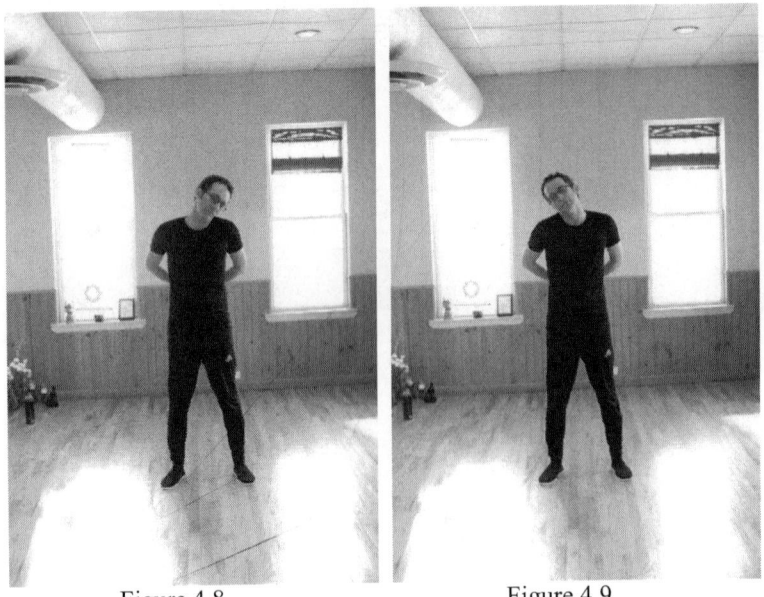

Figure 4.8

Figure 4.9

Picking Cherries

In this movement imagine yourself standing underneath a cherry tree picking cherries.

1. Stand with feet shoulder-width apart and lift your hands over your head. Bend your knees and sink your tailbone down.

2. Look and stretch upward first with one hand and then the other to pick the imaginary cherries.

3. Repeat 8 times in each side.

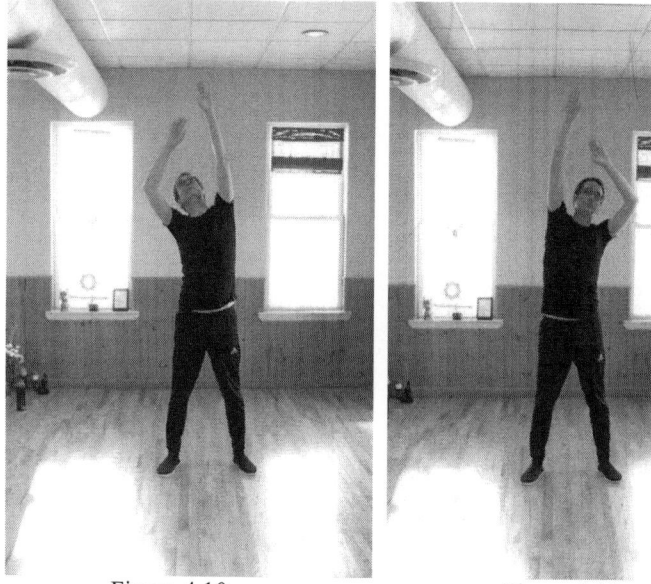

Figure 4.10   Figure 4.11

Beautiful Lady Turns Her Waist

This old Qigong movement helps loosen the hips, lower back and tight muscles. Waist turning is an old remedy for habitual constipation.

1. Stand with your feet facing forward, shoulder-width apart and put your palms on your lower back, over your kidneys (as if you were holding them) or you can also put them on your waist.

2. Keeping your legs straight (if it's hard you can bend your knees a little), rotate your waist in a clockwise direction at a slow, relaxed pace seven times and breathe naturally.

3. Rotate your waist seven times in the opposite direction.

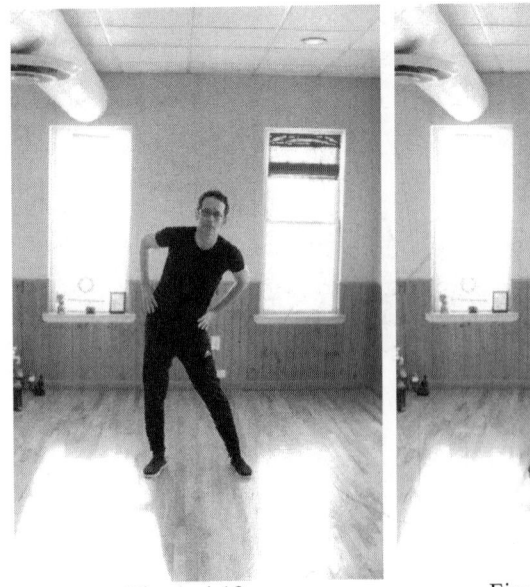

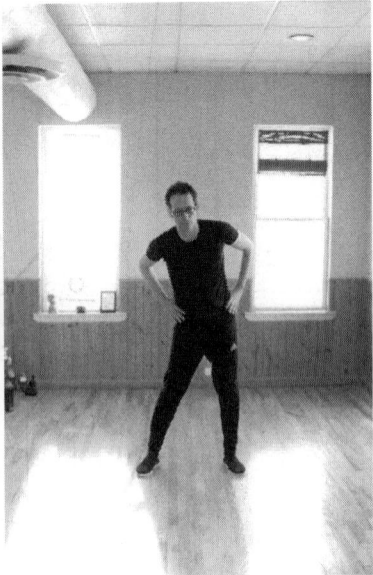

Figure 4.12   Figure 4.13

Spinal Twist

This exercise is beneficial for warming up the center of the body. In this movement you will swing your arms from left to right. While you are twisting, make sure that your head is lifted, that your arms are limp, your hands soft and that your feet are always straight.

1. Stand with feet shoulder-width apart, arms and upper back relaxed. Slowly turn from left to right, rotating from the hips and waist. Allow the momentum from the center of your body to move your arms so they gently knock across the lower back and abdomen.

2. Look over your shoulder as you turn. Make sure your knees are a little bent which will allow more space for movement. As you turn make sure your hips don't sway back and forth. Continue the rotation for 2 minutes.

3. Slowly, naturally unwind and bring your arms back to your sides.

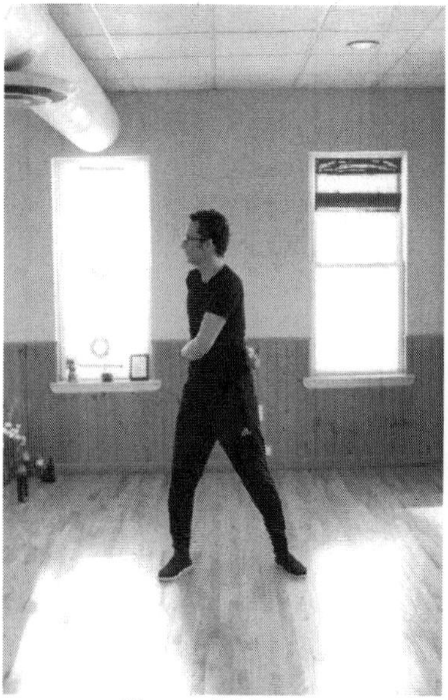

Figure 4.14 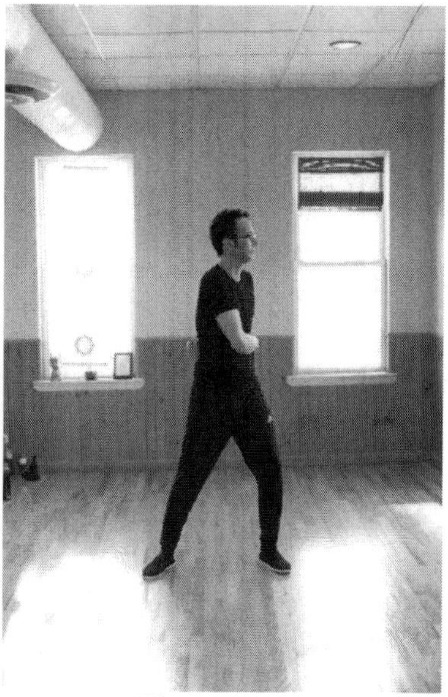   Figure 4.15

Bear Swimming

The arm movements for this exercise are similar to the breast stroke in swimming. This movement can also be done sitting down.

1. Stand with feet shoulder-width apart and palms facing up.

2. Move your hands forward until your arms are almost straight. Turn the palms out so they face away from you.

3. Push the palms outward and circle them around to your sides. Return the palms down and repeat 8 times.

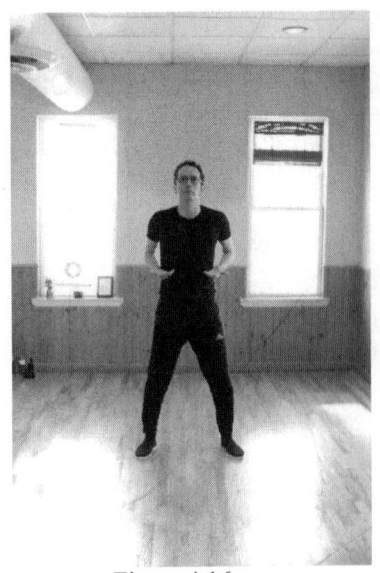

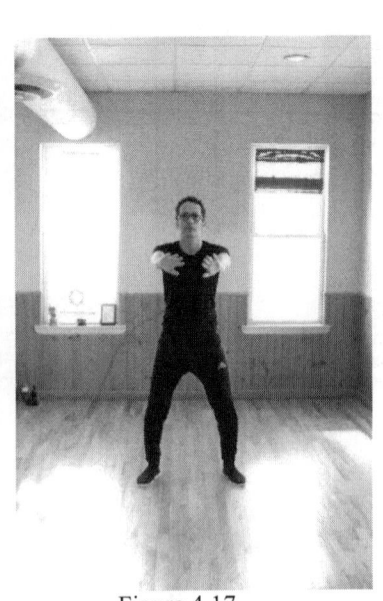

Figure 4.16   Figure 4.17

Lifting the Heels and Opening the Arms

1. Stand with feet shoulder-width apart and arms at your side.

2. Inhale and lift your feet off the ground by rising high on your toes. At the same time lift your arms to the side. Hold for a few seconds and then exhale and lower your feet and palms down.

3. Repeat 8 times.

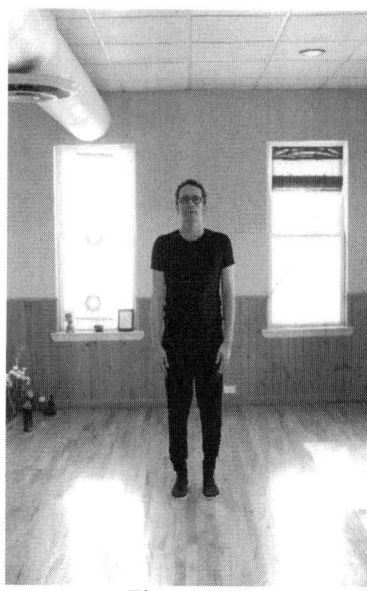

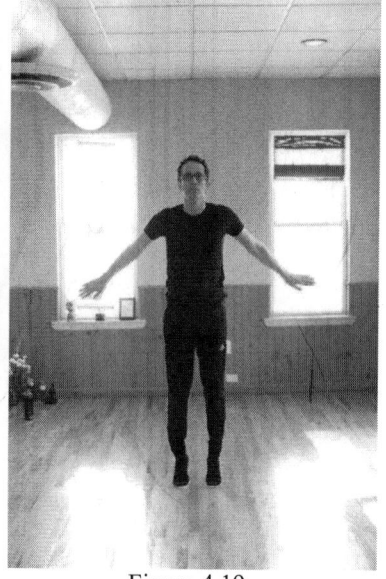

Figure 4.18   Figure 4.19

Full Body Shaking

This movement is good for releasing stress in the body. Keep your body loose throughout the exercise.

1. Begin by shaking your wrists and hands. Next, shake your shoulders and elbows. Then bring movement into the entire body by bouncing up and down on your heels. Keep the head, neck, and shoulders relaxed as you allow the vibration from the shaking to move throughout your body.

2. As you bounce, inhale through the nose and exhale through the mouth. You can shake anywhere between one to three minutes.

3. This movement concludes the set. After you finished it, bring your palms on top of your lower Dantian, stand still and breathe smoothly and slowly for two minutes.

Chapter Five

The Eight Pieces of Brocade

The Ba Duan Jin, which means the "Eight Pieces of Brocade", is very popular and highly regarded for its health-promoting benefits and elegant, graceful movements. There are many theories about the origin and development of the Eight Pieces of Brocade.

Qigong Master Kenneth Cohen comments that the eighth-century Daoist treatise *Xiu Zhen Shi Shu* ("The Ten Treatises on Restoring the Original Vitality"), attributes the development of the Eight Section Brocade to one of the legendary Eight Immortals of Chinese folklore, Chong Li-quan.[16]

Marshal Yue Fei (1103-1142) from the Southern Song Dynasty is said to have created the Eight Pieces of Brocade to improve the health of his soldiers. Yue Fei is one of the most celebrated heroes in the history of China. There is no evidence, however, to support this version. Most likely his name was attached to the Eight Pieces to give them more popular lineage.

There are many names and variations of the Eight Pieces, as is the case in many Qigong movements. So you might find different names to these movements in other books, but the intent in all of them and the basic principles are the same. There are both seated and standing versions of the Eight Pieces. This book will only present the standing one.

Ba Duan Jin is great for beginners. Although simple, these exercises have a lot to offer. Repeat each individual "piece of brocade" 6 to 8 times.

---

[16] Cohen. *The Way of Qigong*. P, 186.

Piece 1: Double Hands Hold Up the Heavens

This movement works especially with the "triple burner" (three parts of the body: lower, middle, upper). This piece benefits the lungs, the heart, the spine, the back and helps digestion.

1. Stand with legs shoulder-width apart, palms facing your legs. Raise your palms, facing upward and as you inhale, interlace your fingers in front of your body and slowly lift the fingers upward. Turn the palms towards the heavens and stretch up.

2. Lift your head up and look at your fingers. Now lower it back down so you are looking straight ahead. Keep your mind calm.

3. Slowly unlace the fingers and lower your palms as you inhale sinking your knees down, switching to exhalation as you reach the level of your heart.

4. Complete the piece by returning your hands to your sides.

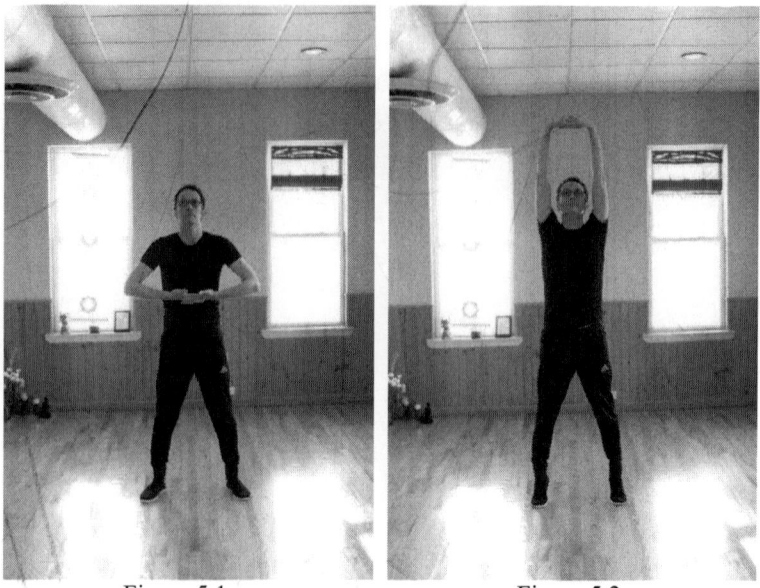

Figure 5.1   Figure 5.2

Piece 2: Pulling the Bow to Shoot the Arrow

This movement is used to strengthen the kidneys, shoulders, chest, arms and lungs. Make sure when you take a wide stance you keep your back straight and tuck the tailbone.

1. Take a wide stance. Bend your knees in the "horse-riding" position. If you are flexible, try to widen the stance with the thighs parallel to the ground (your stance will improve with time).

2. Inhale as you cross your arms, left arm across your chest and right arm crossing your chest over your left arm.

3. Exhale as you "pull the bow to shoot the arrow." Pull your right elbow back high, to your chest level as if you are pulling a string on a bow to shot an arrow. The index finger and thumb of the front hand are extended with the three remaining fingers closed into the palm. Look through your extended index finger and thumb as if you were looking far away.

4. Switch position by turning in the opposite direction while inhaling, crossing your arms again before executing the movement.

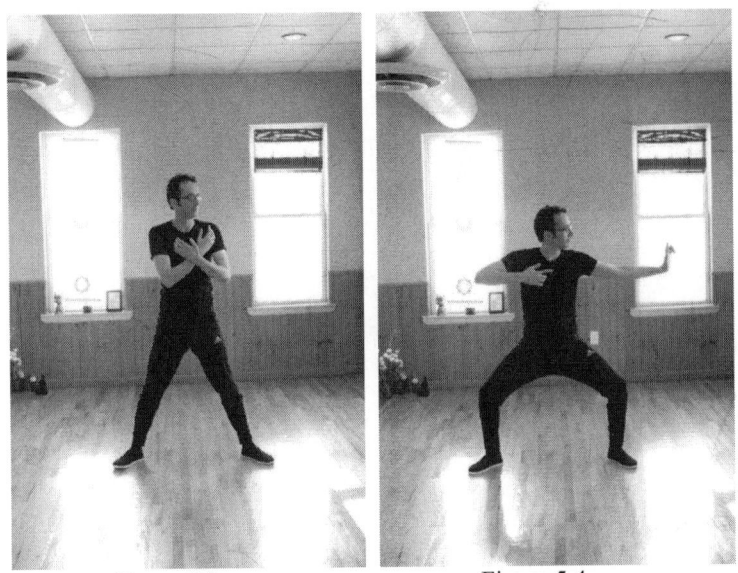

Figure 5.3   Figure 5.4

5. Complete the piece by inhaling as you cross your arms and raise your body up, then exhaling as you return your arms to your sides.

Piece 3: Raise the Arms to Regulate the Spleen (Separating Heaven and Earth)

This movement works on the stomach; it also stretches the torso and the upper back. This up and down palm push improves the Qi circulation in the liver and spleen. If you wish, you can sink your knees as you switch from side to side.

1. Stand with feet shoulder-width apart, arms by your sides. Inhale as you cross your arms in front of your chest.

2. Exhale as you raise the right palm above your head and at the same time push the left palm down, maintaining curvature in the arms.

3. Switch palms and repeat on the opposite side. Don't tense the muscles; try to move in a relaxed way.

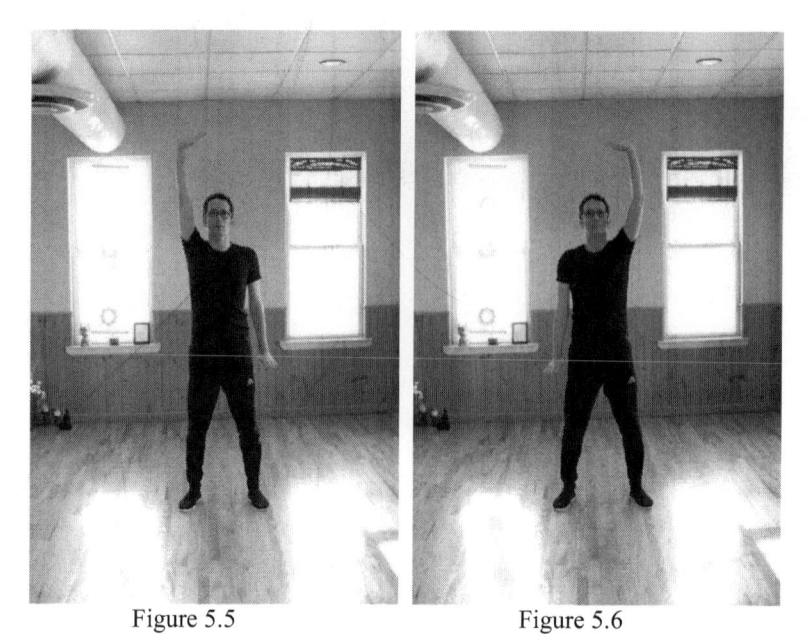

Figure 5.5

Figure 5.6

Piece 4: The Wise Owl Gazes Backward

This movement improves vision, fatigue and distress. It's also good for neck and shoulder tensions, which are common areas where we hold stress.

1. Begin with feet shoulder-width apart, arms resting naturally at your sides, palms facing your legs. Inhale as you raise your palms, facing upward while bending your knees.

2. Slowly turn the head and look to the left side as far as you can without straining your neck. Push your hands downward, straightening your legs while extending your spine. Then return your head to the front as you inhale.

3. Inhale as you move to repeat this sequence on the right side. Complete the piece by exhaling as your arms return to your sides.

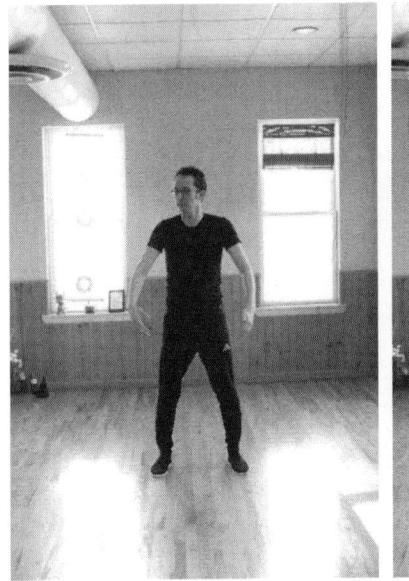

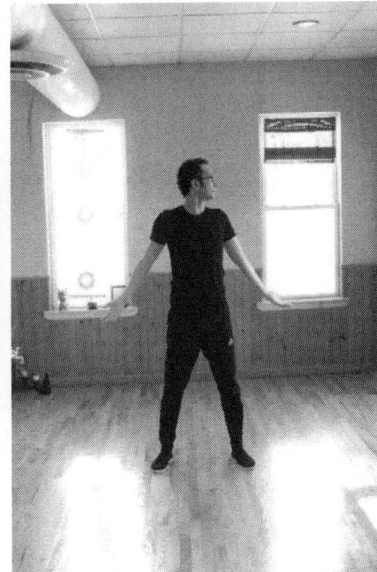

Figure 5.7   Figure 5.8

Piece 5: Bending Over and Wagging the Tail

Bending the head and the body forward from side to side loosens up the lungs and excess Qi (heart fire, according to the five element theory). It also increases the flexibility of the spine and strengthens the low back, hips and thighs.

1. Take a wide stance. If you are flexible try to widen your stance with the thighs parallel to the ground, hands resting on your thighs.

2. Inhale while upright and then exhale as you sway your head and body to the right thigh in a diagonal side motion. And then back up to center with a straight back. Try to maintain a straight back as you sway your body. Also strive to bend from your hips, not from your back.

3. Repeat the move in the opposite direction.

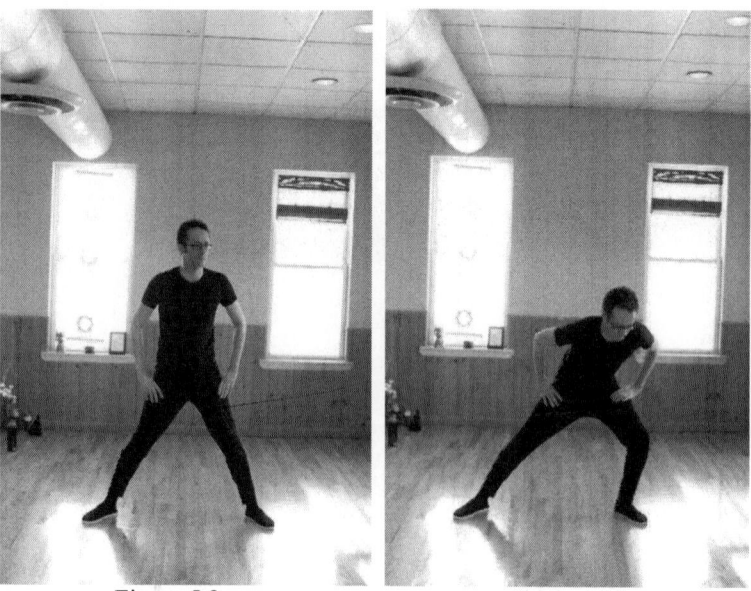

Figure 5.9   Figure 5.10

Piece 6: Two Hands Hold the Feet to Strengthen the Kidneys

This movement is good for the lower back and the hamstrings. As the title of the piece suggests, the movement strengthens the kidneys.

1. Begin with feet shoulder-width apart. Inhale and press both hands up in front of your chest all the way until they reach above you head with the palm facing down. Stay and breathe for a few seconds.

2. Then bend forward (if you have back problems don't bend too much) and trace your hands around your waist to your lower back/kidney area. While moving let your hands slide down to your low back and the backs of your legs, ultimately bringing your hands in front of your feet. If you wish you can touch the toes.

3. Begin to inhale as you lift your arms in front of you, palms out, and bring your body back to an upright position.

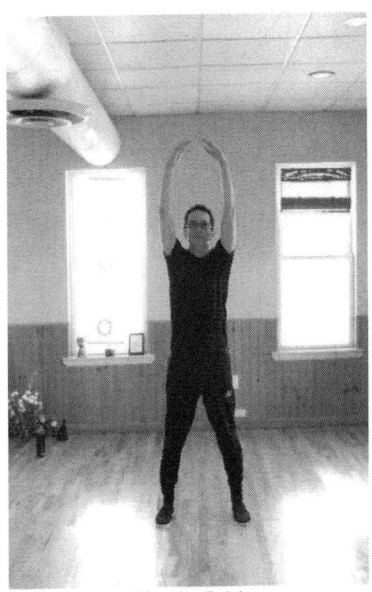

Figure 5.11   Figure 5.12

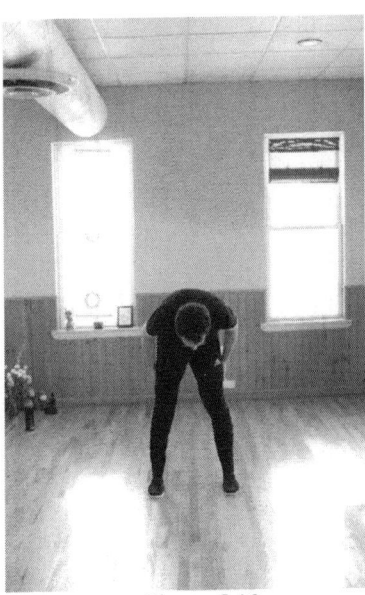

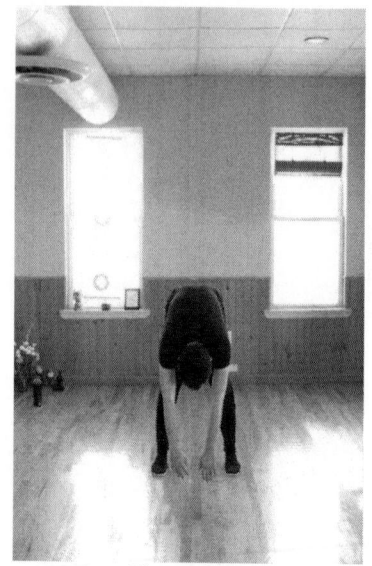

Figure 5.13

Piece 7: Punching With Angry Eyes

As the title says this movement is done with an intent gaze. It releases pent up anger and frustration. By sinking your legs in this movement you will build strength in your upper back, legs and arms.

1. Take a wide stance and bend your knees, similar to the second piece. Pull both hands in with arms around chest level. The hand movement is a little complicated. Bring the thumbs into the palms and form your hands into lightly clenched upright fists by your sides. Your elbows should be pulled back.

2. Exhale as you slowly extend your right arm forward and spiral your fist in front of your body with the clenched palm facing downward. Open the fist, so the palm faces out and the thumb is pointing down. Rotate the wrist so the palm is facing up. Bring the thumb back into the center of the palm and close four fingers on top of the thumb. Don't lock your elbow joint.

3. At the completion of the punch, begin to inhale as you pull your right hand and elbow back to your side and before you exhale while slowly punching out with your left hand.

4. Complete the piece by inhaling as you raise your body up, exhaling as you lower your hands to your sides.

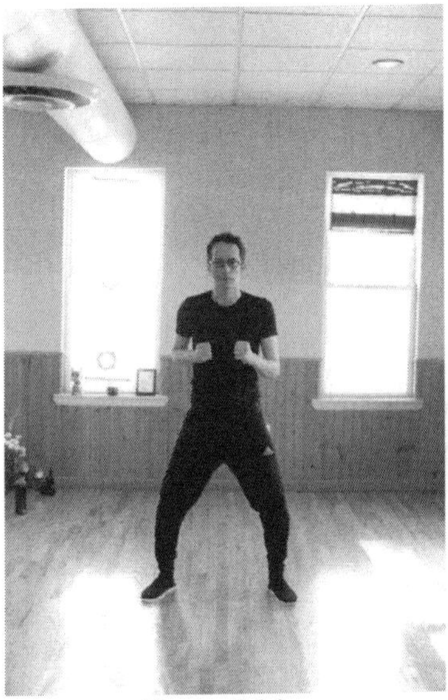

Figure 5.14

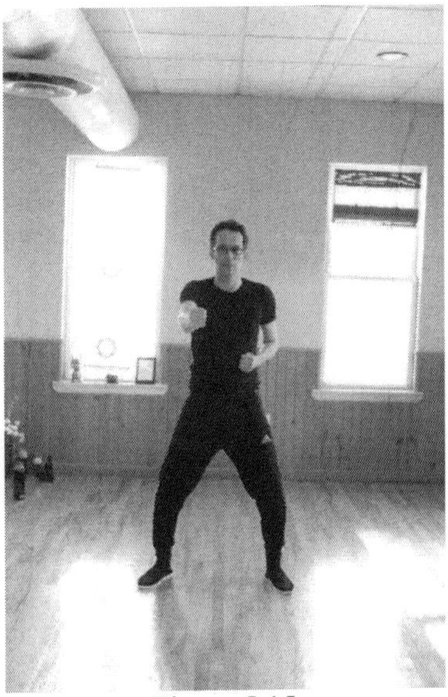

Figure 5.15

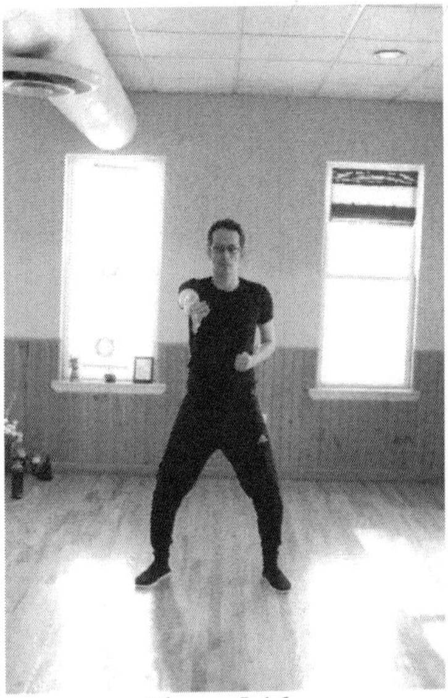

Figure 5.16

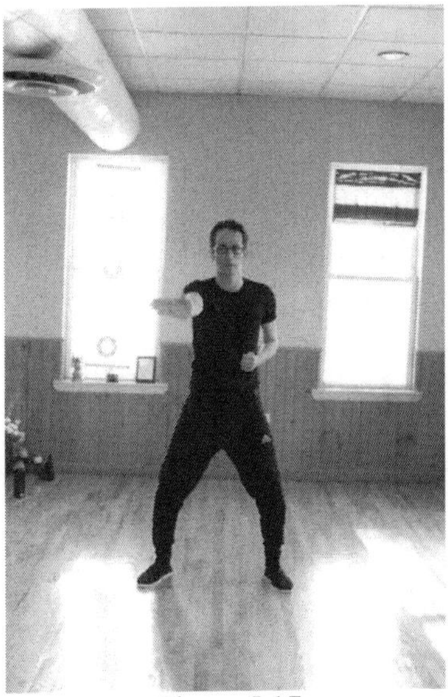

Figure 5.17

Piece 8: Bouncing on Heels to Shake off Stress and Illness

This movement is the easiest and simplest piece of the set. It strengthens the ankles and calves. If you wish, you can raise your palms, facing upward while doing this movement.

1. Your feet should be close to one another and arms at your side. Keep your mind calm.

2. Inhale, push your head up and lift your feet off the ground by rising high on your toes. Hold for a few seconds and then exhale and lower your feet down.

3. This movement concludes the set. After you finish it, bring your palms on top of your lower Dantian, stand still and breathe smoothly and slowly for two minutes.

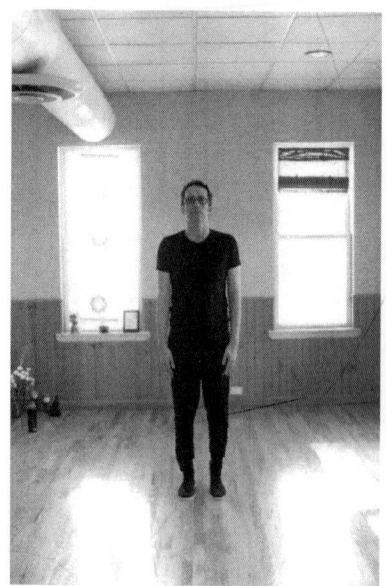

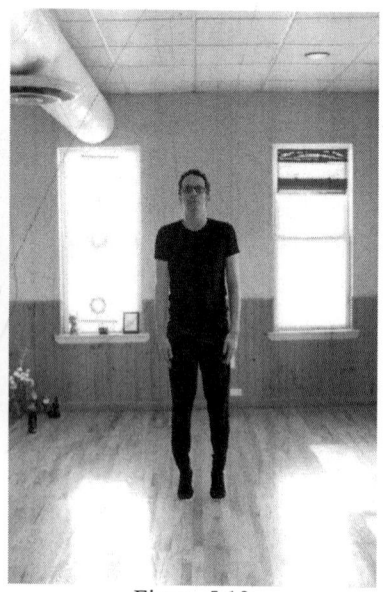

Figure 5.18   Figure 5.19

Chapter Six

Tai Chi Qigong 18 Movements

"You must be shapeless, formless, like water.
When you pour water in a cup, it becomes the cup.
When you pour water in a bottle, it becomes the bottle.
When you pour water in a teapot, it becomes the teapot.
Water can drip and it can crash. Become like water my friend."

Bruce Lee

Tai Chi Qigong 18 series was created in Shanghai, China, by Professor Lin Hou Sheng. Set one, 18 movements (Shibashi) were created in 1979. Master Lin created several other routines through the years. The routine presented in this book (set number 1) combines movements from the Yang style Tai Chi and Qigong exercises. Many movements have names commonly used in the Tai Chi forms.[17]

Practice Guidelines

Relax deeply while standing with your feet firmly rooted to the floor, knees slightly bent. Breathe using slow, continuous breaths. Place your tongue lightly at the roof of your mouth, behind your teeth. Move your body with the lightest of effort, as if you were "moving in water." Repeat each individual movement six to eight times. Try to find a slow pace for these movements. Shibashi form is suitable for persons of all ages.

---

[17] Chris Jarmey. *The Theory and Practice of Taiji Qigong*. Berkley: North Atlantic Books, 2005.

Movement 1: Opening the Door (Open Tai Chi)

"Opening the Door," is the name of the first movement, it also commences most Tai Chi routines.
This is one of the simplest Tai Chi and Qigong exercises. In this movement, you will move the body up and down with the breath. Let the body rise up with the in breath and then soften and relax the body with the out breath.

1. Begin with feet shoulder-width apart, hands at waist, palms down. Inhale and lift your arms up in front of your body until they are about shoulder height.

2. Slowly exhale and sink down your arms until your hands are around waist level, slightly bending and softening your knees.

3. Repeat seven times.

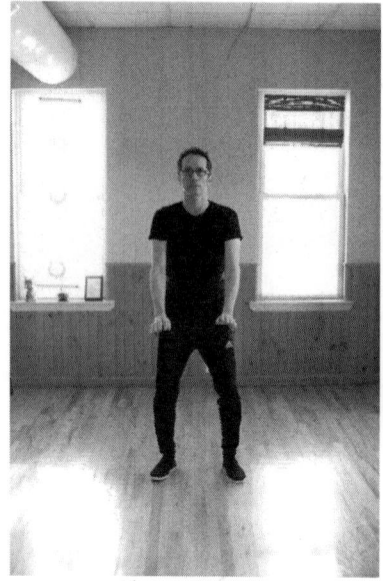

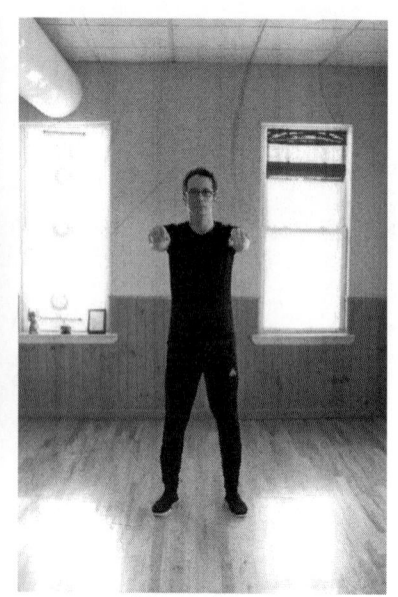

Figure 6.1   Figure 6.2

Movement 2: Opening the Chest

In the second movement we expand the first movement by opening the chest and rotating the palms to face one another. There is spontaneity here, allowing the movement to be natural and unforced. We are not looking to stretch the arms out in a traditional sense but more accurately we are looking for a sense of opening. The movement of gently moving/tilting forwards and back also massages the Yong Quan point on the sole of the foot.

1. Begin with feet shoulder-width apart, inhale and lift your arms up in front of your body, until they are about shoulder height.

2. Turn palms facing each other. Exhale and move your hands away from each other, arms fully extended to sides.

3. Inhale and bring your arms back together until your hands are shoulder-width apart with the palms facing one another.

4. Then exhale slowly and lower your arms until your hands are around waist level with knees slightly bent. Repeat seven times.

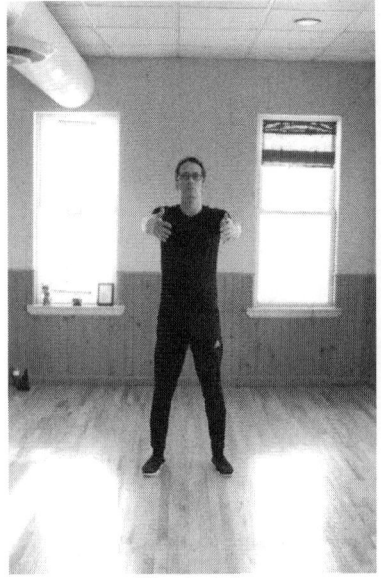

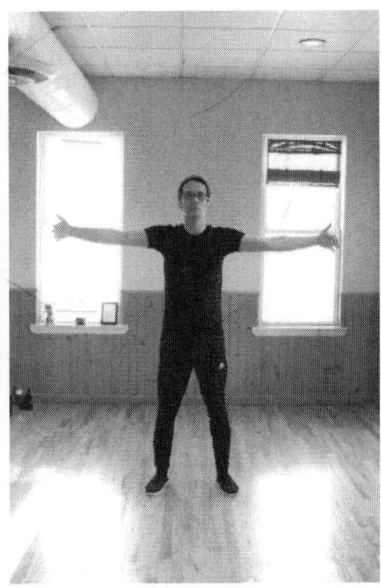

Figure 6.3   Figure 6.4

Movement 3: Rainbow Dance

In this movement you will turn your head from side to side while covering the crown of your head with your other hand. You will also connect Qi energy points Lao Gong from your hand to Bai Hui, which is on top of your head.

1. Begin with your feet a little wider than shoulder-width apart. Now transfer the weight to the right leg, putting all of your weight into it. Keep knees slightly bent.

2. At the same time extend left arm out to left side at shoulder height, looking at the open palm. Raise your right hand and hold it above your head with the Lao Gong point facing the top of your head (Bai Hui point).

3. Begin gently shifting your weight to the left leg as you move your arms in a flowing way above your head. Keep knees slightly bent and extend right arm out to right side at shoulder height. The left palm faces down above center of head.

4. Repeat six times (three times each side).

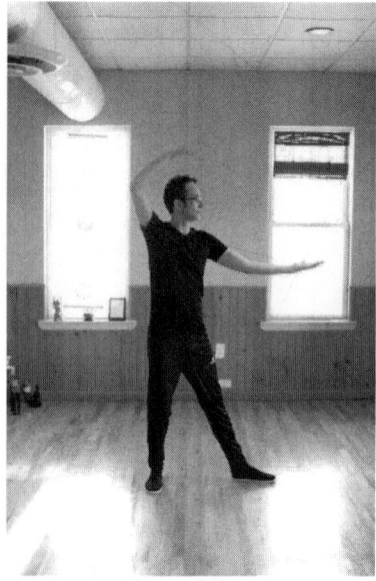

Figure 6.5   Figure 6.6

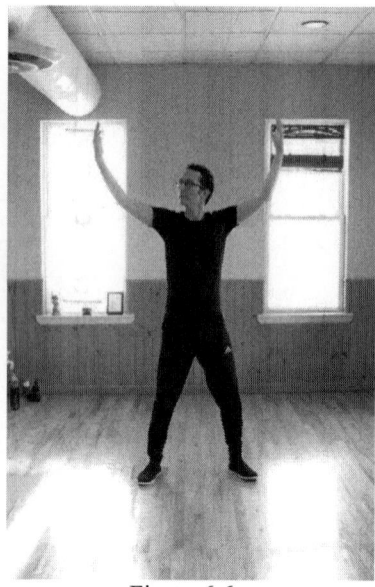

Movement 4: Separating the Clouds

This movement is great for extending the breath, stress relief and for relaxation. Try to coordinate the breath, inhaling as you raise your palms and exhaling as you lower your hands.

1. Stand with legs shoulder-width apart and bring your hands in front of your Dantian, palms facing up.

2. As you inhale deeply, move your hands all the way over your head, keeping the elbows soft, and cross hands left over right at wrist.

3. On the exhale, separate your palms and turn them away from you, circling them down and around to either side of your body, bringing them to rest again at the Dantian.

4. Repeat seven times.

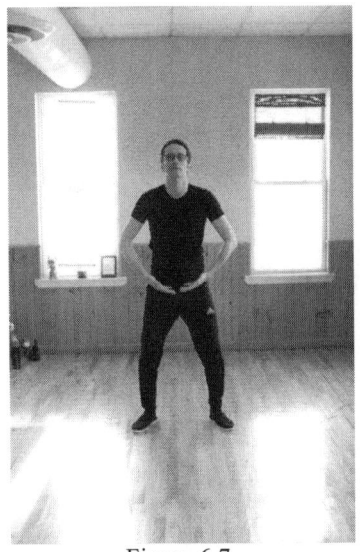

Figure 6.7   Figure 6.8

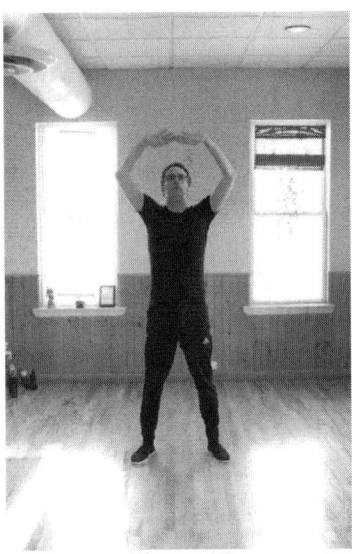

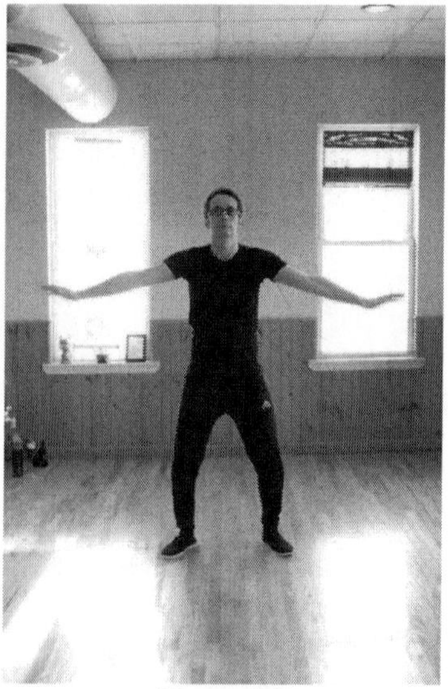

Figure 6.9

Movement 5: Repulse the Monkey

The full Chinese name of this movement is "dao nian hou." Dao means backward, nian means to repel away and hou is monkey. In the Tai Chi form it's done while walking backwards. In this form it's done without the walking.

1. Begin with feet shoulder-width apart, inhale and lift your left hand extended in front of the body, palm upward at chest height, right hand out to the side at shoulder height, palm upward.

2. Turn from your hips and waist area. Push the right hand forward and down, withdrawing your left hand so that the palms cross in front of your body. Exhale as you turn your waist to the left to transfer your weight to your right leg.

3. Push your left hand forward and draw the right hand back. Transfer your weight to your other foot as you turn your waist in the opposite direction.

4. Repeat six times (three times each side).

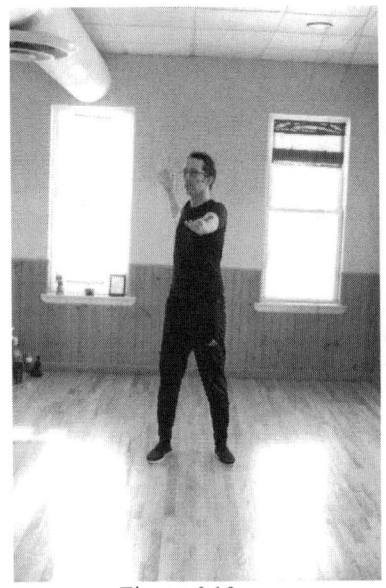

Figure 6.10   Figure 6.11

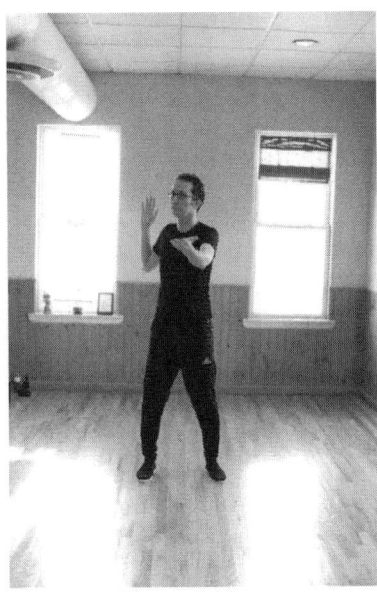

Movement 6: Rowing the Boat in the Centre of the Lake

This movement is good for the kidneys and for stress. It's also good for the lower back.

1. Begin with feet shoulder-width apart, inhale, reach back both palms behind your head and look backwards.

2. Now move your hands forward like you are rowing a boat and gently bend your knees. Draw your hands back to Dantian.

3. Repeat, lean back and lift your palms up in a wide circle, straightening your legs slightly.

4. Repeat seven times.

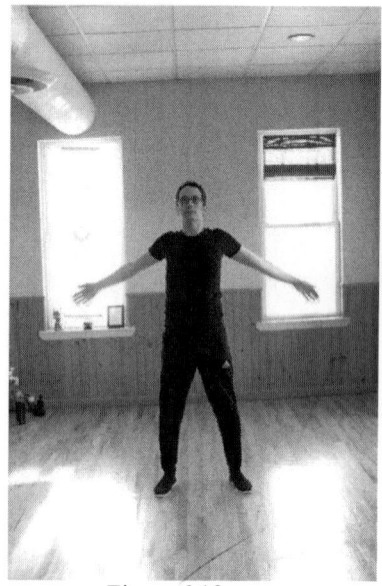

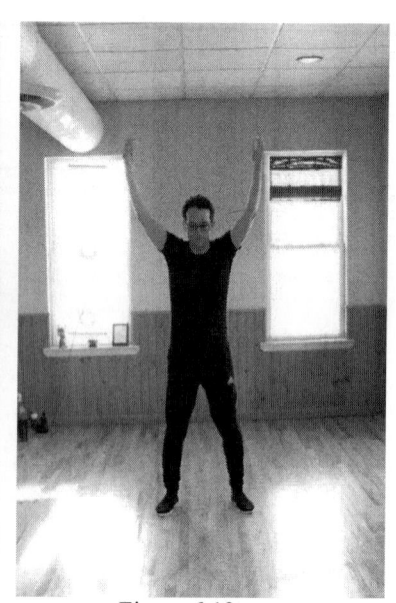

Figure 6.12   Figure 6.13

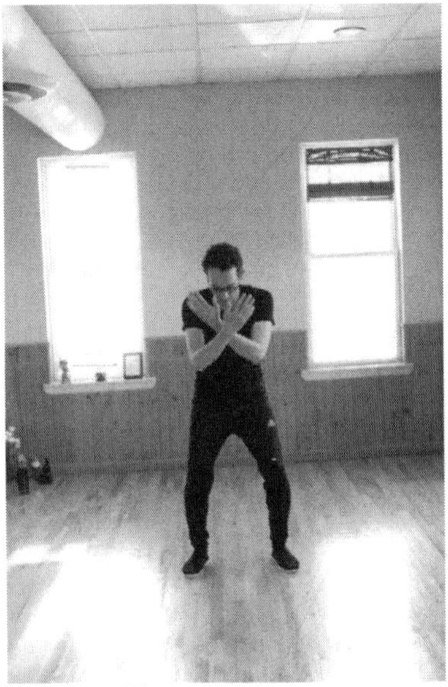

Figure 6.14

Movement 7: Lifting the Ball

This exercise is more dynamic. You lift off your heel and lift your arms from side to side. Try to find your own internal rhythm as you move from side to side.

1. Begin with feet shoulder-width apart, inhale and shift your weight onto your left leg, allowing the heel of the right leg to come off the ground. As you turn to the left and bring the right palm up to the left above shoulder height. Imagine as if you are really lifting a ball or holding a tea cup. Look to where you are reaching.

2. Keep your left arm by your side and move your weight into your left leg. The right leg then stretches on tiptoe with the heel up. Turn the waist and inhale.

3. Change from one side to the other, breathing in on the upward movement and out on the down.

4. Repeat six times (three times each side).

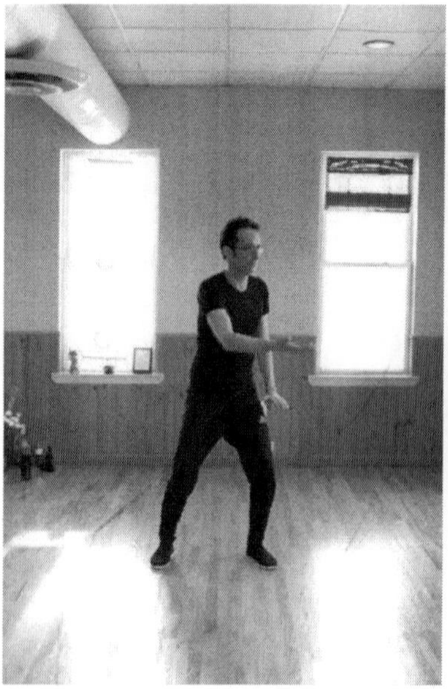

Figure 6.15 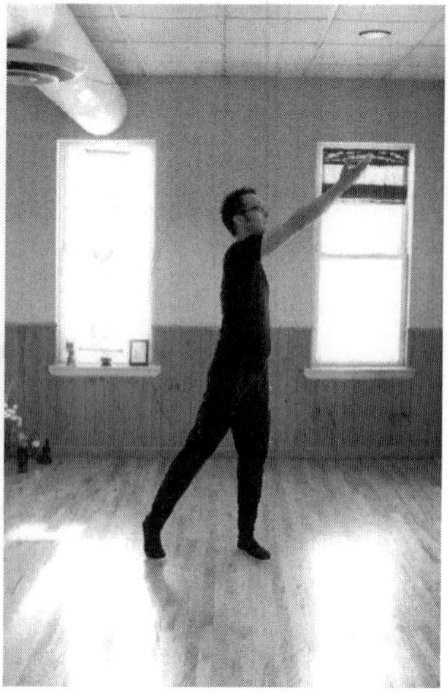   Figure 6.16

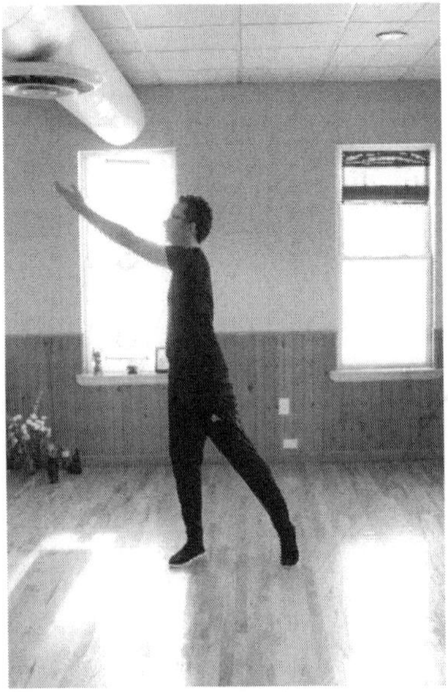

Figure 6.17

Movement 8: Looking at the Moon

This movement, like the previous one, is also very dynamic and light. It's similar to lifting the ball but this one is done by looking backward into the moon.

1. Begin with feet shoulder-width apart, inhale and turn your body backward toward the left side, shifting your weight into your left leg, raising the heel of your right foot. At the same time look in the direction of your hands and imagine you are looking at the moon.

2. Exhale and twist the body, allowing your knees to bend, and shift your weight into the right foot, raising the heel of your left foot. Allow a nice swiping movement.

3. Repeat six times (three times each side).

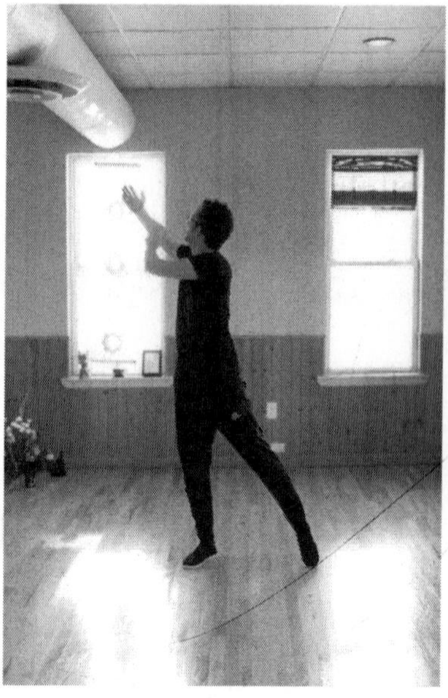

Figure 6.18 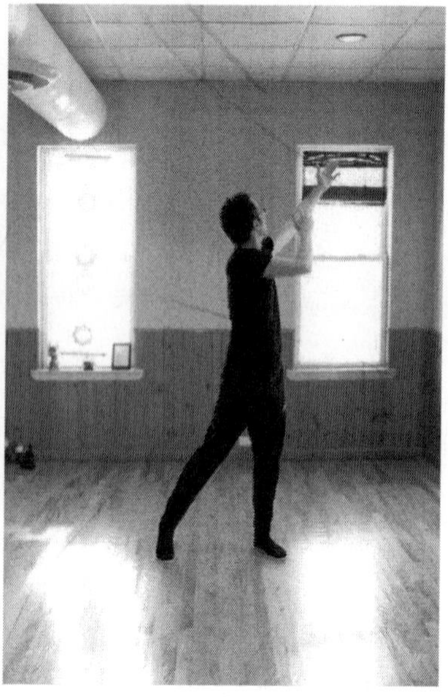   Figure 6.19

Movement 9: Turning the Waist and Pushing the Palms

In this exercise you will be pushing your hand across your body to the opposite corner and then pulling your other hand back.

1. Begin with feet shoulder-width apart, inhale and take your left arm behind you looking to the back, palm facing down (Hegu about chest height).

2. At the same time push your right palm out in front of you (fully extending your arm) as you turn your waist to the left and exhale. Look behind and push palm from left side to the right side.

3. Repeat seven times.

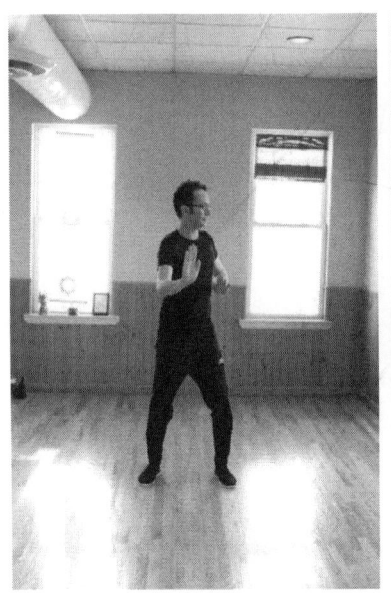

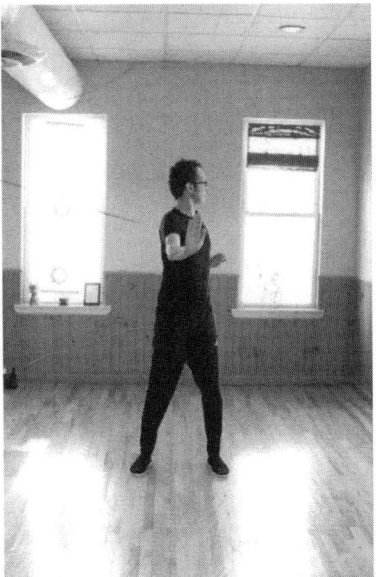

Figure 6.20   Figure 6.21

Movement 10: Cloud Hands in a Horse-Riding Stance

The Chinese name of this movement is "yun shou" and means cloud hands. The movement is done like the name implies- by waving your hands like floating clouds. In different styles of Tai Chi (Chen, Yang and Wu) Cloud hands is performed in many different ways, usually by walking sideways, while in this form it's done in horse stance. If you only have time to practice one move for health, cloud hands should be it. Practicing this movement will enhance your coordination.

1. Feet are slightly separated beyond shoulder-width, the knees are slightly bent.
2. Move the right arm clockwise, with palm facing the body, and left palm is at waist level facing the right palm. Imagine as if you are holding a big ball.
3. Allow your right palm to circle down and the left palm to rise up. Turn your body from the waist and allow the arms to follow turn.
4. Repeat the process by swapping the hands again and turning the waist from left side to right side.

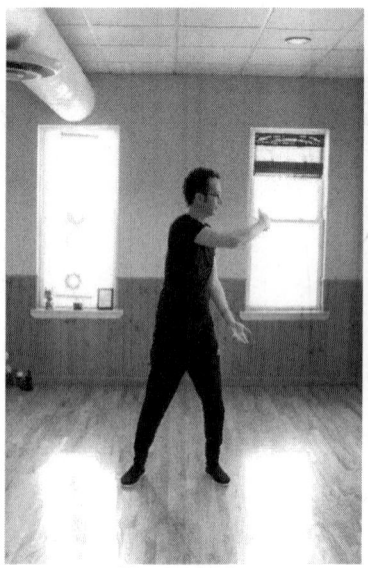

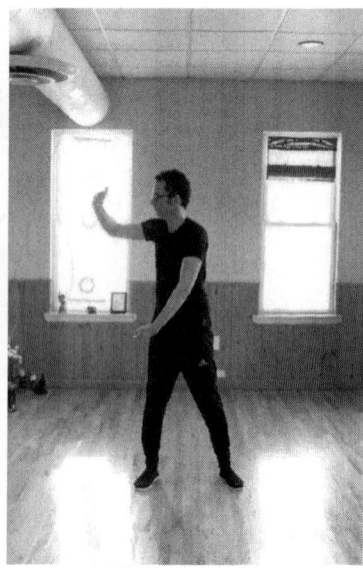

Figure 6.22   Figure 6.23

Movement 11: Scooping the Sea and Looking at the Sky. Touching the Sea

This movement is done in bow stance. You will bend down as if you are scooping something from the floor. This movement is excellent for the lower back and helps strengthen the legs.

1. Begin in bow stance, feet about shoulder-width apart, with the right foot forwards and the left foot at the back turned out at about 45 degrees. Begin with your weight in the back (right) leg and then extend arms out and up to shoulder height, elbows slightly bent, palms facing forwards.

2. Exhale and shift your weight towards the front (right) leg, at the same time, lean forwards and downwards, lowering your arms down in front of you until they cross hands left over right, just below your (right) knee. Imagine you are scooping from the sea.

3. Inhale as you straighten body upright, opening your arms as you go back. Repeat six time times and then change sides.

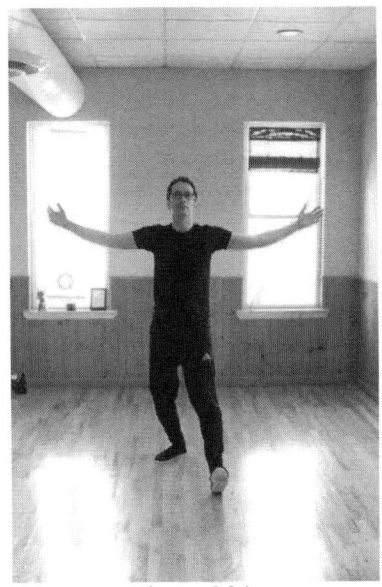

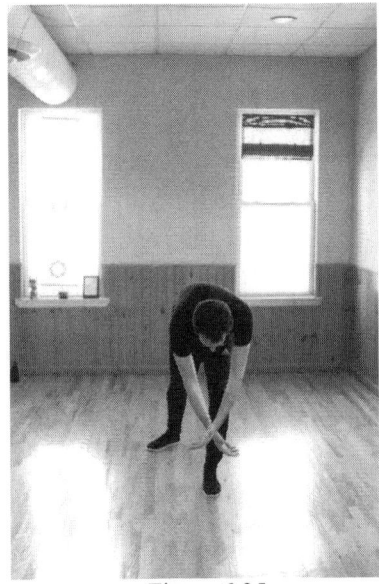

Figure 6.24

Figure 6.25

Movement 12: Pushing the Waves

In this exercise we will connect Hegu point (hand) and Yun Men point (chest). Exhale pushing forwards, inhale and sink back. Try to flow like a wave in this movement, a wave that's going up and down. This exercise strengthens the chest and the lungs.

1. Begin in bow stance, feet about shoulder-width apart. Lift both hands to shoulder height, bringing them towards your chest, so that the Hegu and Yun Men points face one another.

2. Push palms forward (with Lao Gong point open forward) as you bend into the front knee, keeping the weight into the front leg (knee is about 90 degrees). Allow the back leg to be straight.

3. As you return, draw back your fingers into about chest height, sink into the back knee and raise your toes in the front foot. Allow the movement to be smooth.

4. As with the previous movement, repeat six time times, then change sides.

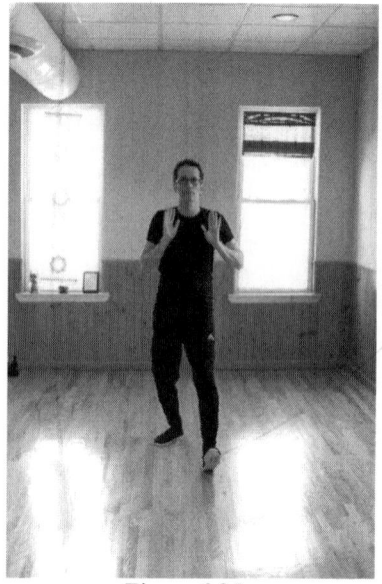

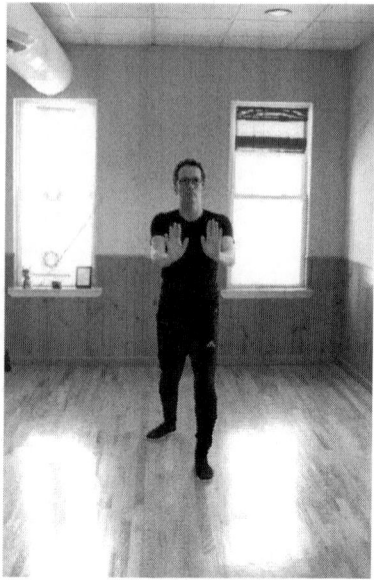

Figure 6.25   Figure 6.26

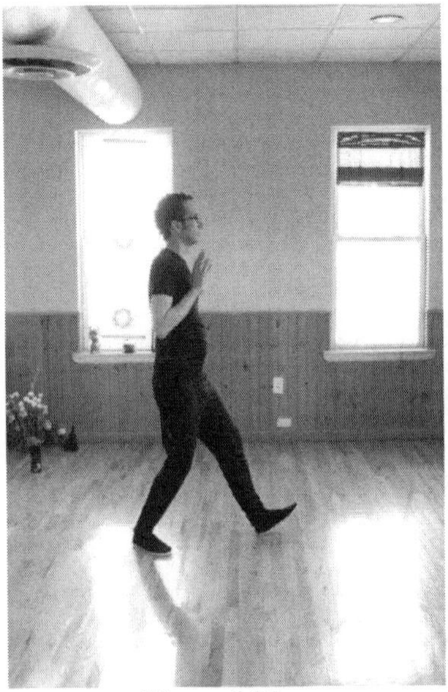

Figure 6.27 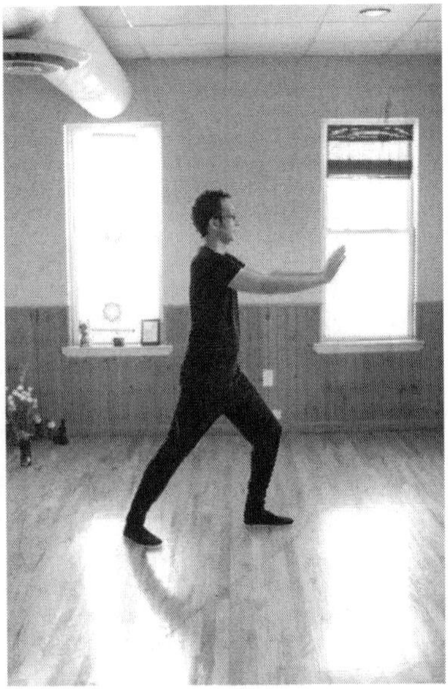   Figure 6.28

Movement 13: Flying Pigeon

This movement, like the previous one is done in bow stance. You will exhale pushing forwards, inhale and sink back. Your arms and chest will open as we move forward and close as we move backwards.

1. Begin in bow stance, feet about shoulder-width apart. Inhale and open your arms out to the side about shoulder height, palms facing forwards.

2. Exhale and shift your weight forward, bending into the front knee, closing your arms as the weight comes into your front leg. Lift the toes of the front leg off the ground as you sink back.

3. As with the previous movement, repeat six time times, then change sides.

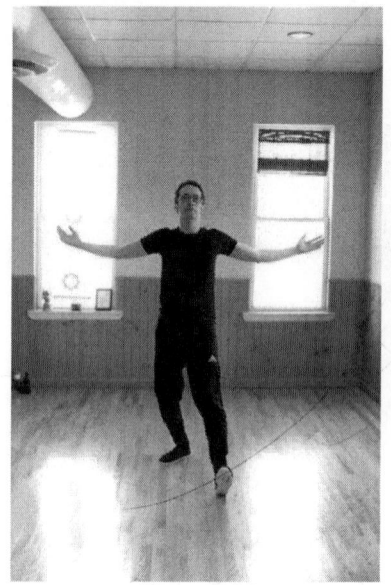

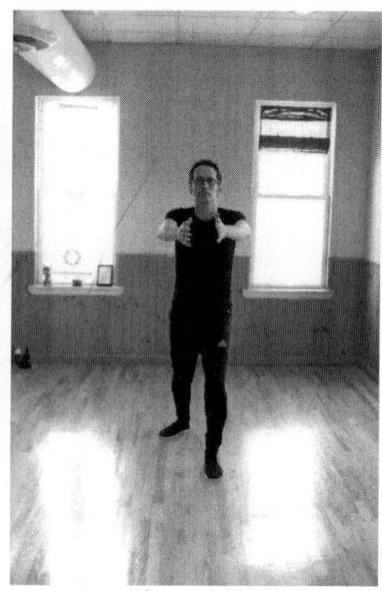

Figure 6.29   Figure 6.30

Movement 14: Punching

In this movement you will punch from waist level, with a vertical fist and thumb up. This exercise strengthens the legs and if you sink down the leg, it is also good for the lungs and breathing. Try to keep your shoulders relaxed, punch softly, don't force it and don't lock the elbows.

1. Begin with feet shoulder-width apart, knees relaxed and soft but not fully bent. Take your hands to your waist, palms up and make loose fists. Your thumb should be on top.

2. Using whole body movement, starting with the right hand, exhale and punch slowly forward and turn the fist around (like a screwdriver) until you have a straight elbow in front of you. Now inhale and bring the hand back to waist level again.

3. Repeat the punch with the left hand, six times.

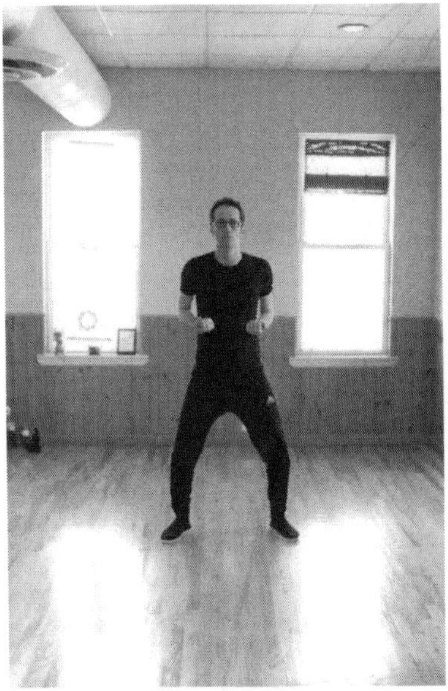

Figure 6.31 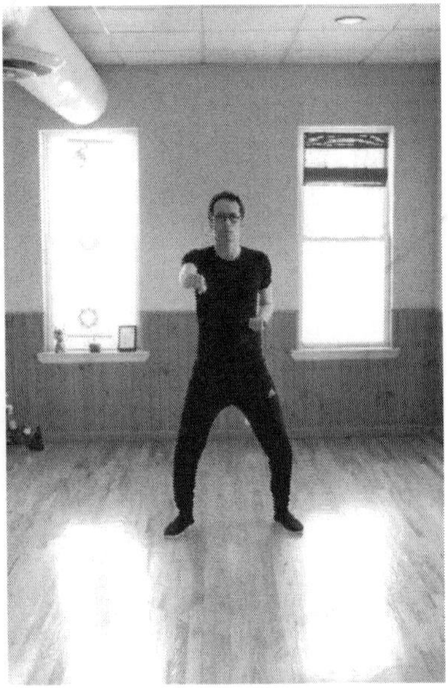   Figure 6.32

Movement 15: Flying Wild Goose

Like many Qigong or Tai Chi movements, this movement imitates an animal. As the name suggests, in this movement you should imagine you are a wild goose flapping its wings up and down.

1. Begin with feet shoulder-width apart, inhale and lift your arms to the sides from the shoulder followed by the elbows, wrists and fingers until your arms are above your shoulders. Your finger tips should be pointing up.

2. Exhale and allow your arms to come down from the shoulder, elbows, wrists and fingers, bending your knees slightly as you lower the arms.

3. Repeat seven times.

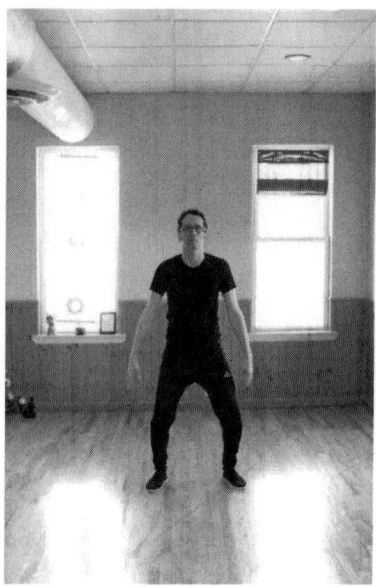

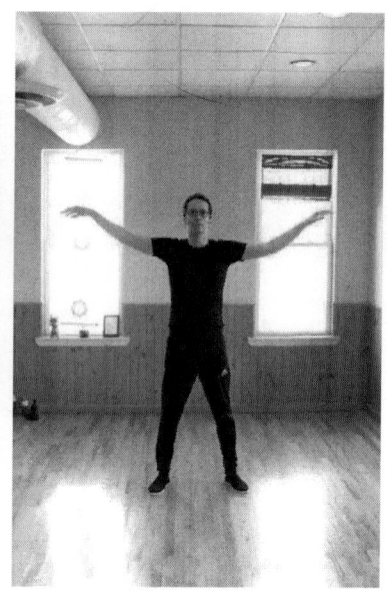

Figure 6.33   Figure 6.34

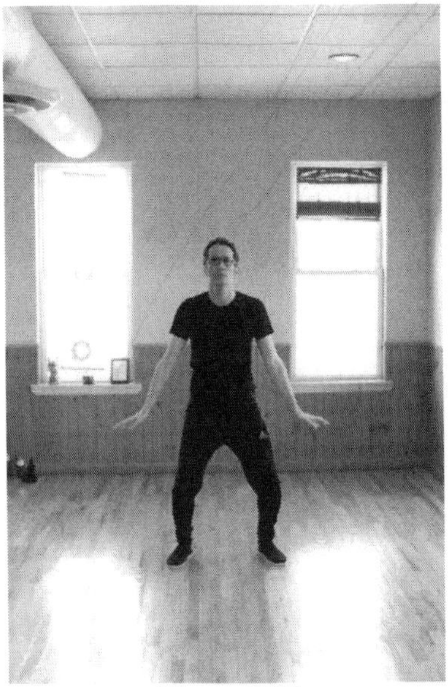

Figure 6.35

Movement 16: Turning like a Wheel

In this movement we make circles with the arms, while turning our hips. This exercise strengthens the back, hips and the waist. Take care with this movement, making sure you are moving slowly and never overstretching. With time this movement will get easier and become fun.

1. Begin with feet shoulder-width apart, inhale and lift the hands on top of your head (connecting to Bai Hui), imagining you are holding a big ball. You will turn right to the side, stretching down all the way to the ground.

2. Scoop the hands across the floor, rotate the hands over and reach out the hand to the sky.

3. Repeat three time times, then rotate from the other direction.

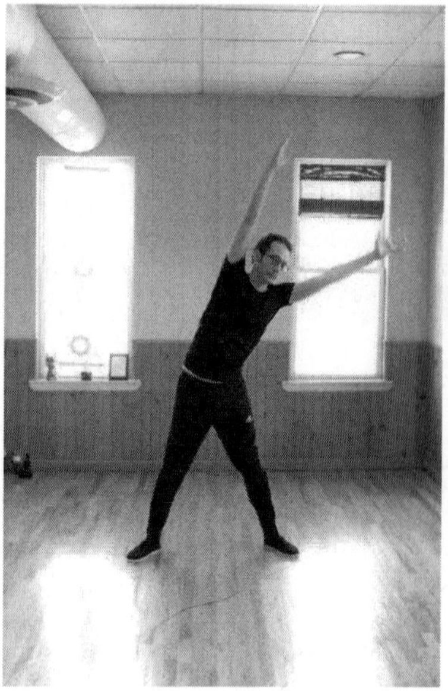

Figure 6.36 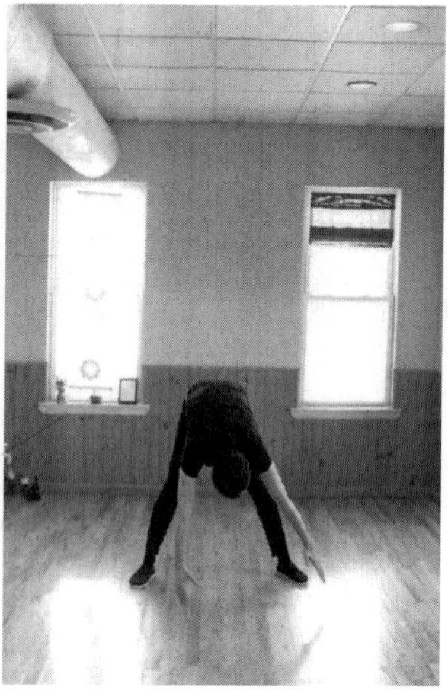   Figure 6.37

Movement 17: Marching and Bouncing a Ball

This is a great balance, coordination and focus exercise. As we get older we start losing our balance. In this movement we are like a puppet on strings with the arm connected to the opposite knee. So when the left arm goes up, the right knee comes up and your right arm is connected to your left knee.

1. Begin with feet shoulder-width apart, inhale and lift your left hand and your left foot at the same time, exhale and release. Your hand should be around shoulder high and knee about 90 degrees.

2. Switch to the other side and lift your right hand and your right foot at the same time. Imagine as if you are lifting the knee with a string in your hand.

3. Another variation of this can be to lift the opposite knee and hand. This will be a great exercise for balance and coordination.

4. Repeat three times on each side.

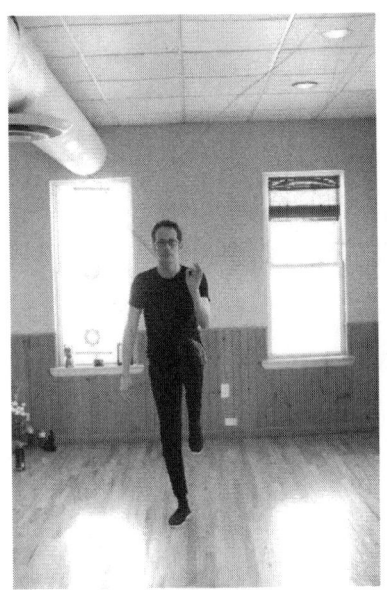

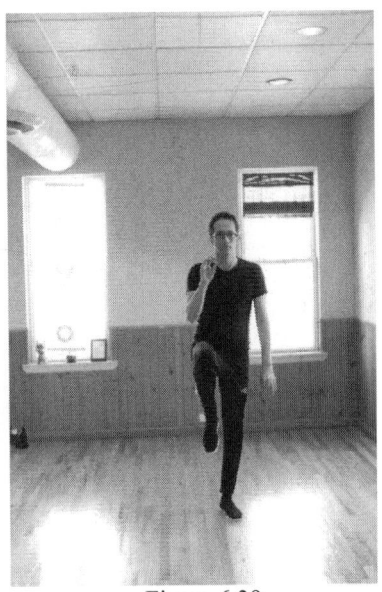

Figure 6.38   Figure 6.39

Movement 18: Balancing the Qi (Sao Gong)

This movement closes the form by bringing the Qi back into the lower Dantian. If you find this movement to be difficult, try it without lifting your heels.

1. Begin with feet shoulder-width apart, palms facing up at about waist height.

2. Inhale and lift your palms to your chest and lift your heels.

3. Exhale and turn the palms down, bring your arms down to your lower Dantian and bring your heels down.

4. Repeat seven times.

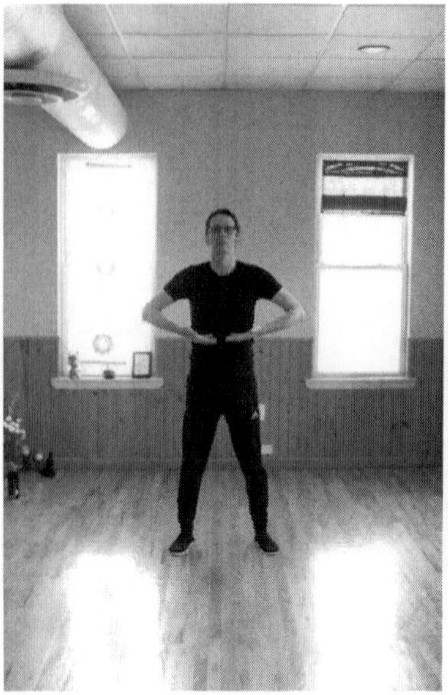

Figure 6.40 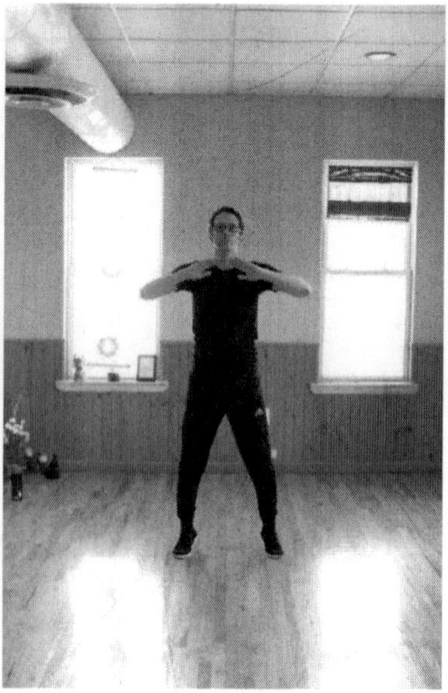   Figure 6.41

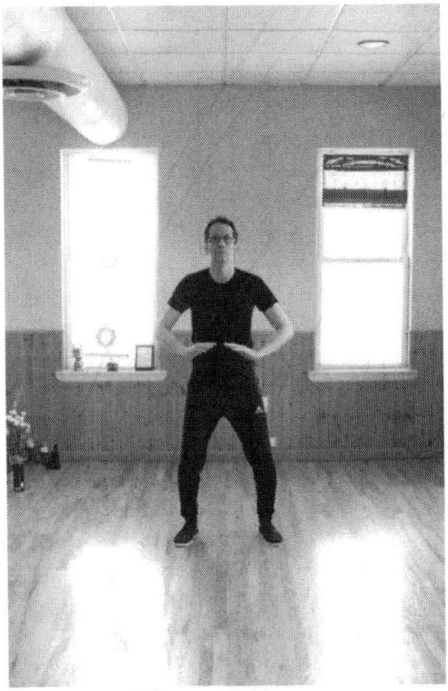

Figure 6.42

Chapter Seven

Qigong for healthy Life Style

"Go with nature and improve what you have."
CK Chu

Healthy Life Style – Nutrition

Qigong and Yoga meditation are very good for healthy and stronger breath but they are also good for digestion. Another source of Qi is the food we eat. Doing Qigong is one aspect of a healthy life style. What we eat is another important aspect. There are hundreds of diet and health books promoting different dietary rules and theories. Both western and eastern diets have their benefits.

Here are some basic tips for healthy eating from a modern perspective:

- Buy and eat local food. That means food that has grown within 500 miles of where you live.

- Buy seasonal food. When I was young strawberries were around for only a few months, but now you can get them all year round. It's better for you to buy seasonal food because it is healthier, cheaper and tastes better.

- Buy local organic vegetables and fruits. Even though organic food tends be more expensive, once in a while try to get some organic vegetables and fruits.

- Fat is good for you! Unsaturated fats are usually the healthier type of fats to eat. They are found in nuts, olive oil, legumes, avocados and oily fishes (such as salmon). Although many diet books will tell you to eat non-fat foods, some fats are good for you in moderation. Just because you eat fat won't make you fat!

- Swap white rice, white flour, white pasta and white bread for whole wheat and whole grains (such as brown rice and whole wheat pasta).

- Try avoiding fast foods and processed foods. Try to cook more and eat out less. When you cook you are more in control of what goes into your food.

- Eat a balanced diet of protein (complete protein includes: fish, eggs, cheese, milk and meat). Protein is essential for growth and repairing of our bodies.

- Buy organic or free range meat. Avoid meats that have hormones or antibiotics. Remember you can buy cheaper cuts such as chicken thighs. Also cutting down on meat is recommended. It takes longer for our digestion system to digest meat. Focus on quality not quantity.

- Eat dairy in moderation. Dairy foods contain nutrients that keep us strong and healthy. The easiest way to add a little dairy to our meal in a balanced way is to serve your meal with a spoonful of yogurt, cheese or ricotta. There are some alternatives to dairy milk such as oat milk, coconut milk or almond milk. These milks have higher calcium than dairy milk.

- Smoothies are always good, due to the fact that we can put many fruits and vegetables in them and they are easier to digest.[18]

- When it comes to eating healthy, the general rule should be: you don't have to be perfect every day, just try to get your balance right across the week. Mix your food to make sure you're eating a varied diet.

---

[18] For more great ideas see Gene Stone. *The Secrets of People Who Never Get Sick,* New York: Workman Publishing Company, 2010.

- Your weekly main meal plan should include: fish once or twice a week, one day poultry, two to three days of meat free meals and very little red meat.

- Eat more vegetables and fruits; they are packed with dietary fiber. They can help you maintain a healthy heart and healthy weight. Try to eat them at every meal and try to eat different colors.

- Eat a big breakfast! This meal is often overlooked but it's so important to give you energy for the rest of your day. It will prevent you from snacking on unhealthy foods throughout your day.

Healthy Eastern Diet Rules

- It's not recommended to eat raw food. Food should be cooked, cooking breaks the food down.

- When it comes to cooking don't deep fry. Try steaming or sautéing. Try eating a variety of foods. Eat more vegetables and less meat.

- Eat slowly and chew your food more. Rather than changing what you eat, according to eastern teachings sometimes you should change the way you eat! Sometimes when we rush we finish our meal in five minutes. It generally takes 20-25 minutes to realize we are full. That's why many people overeat. When you eat slower, more likely you won't over eat.

- Focus on the food while you are eating. In modern times, we multi-task and do several things at the same time. When you are eating it's important to have your full attention on the food you are eating. You need to sit down while you eat and not eat in front of the computer or TV.

- Drink more tea! Tea is one of the many gifts China has brought to the world. Tea promotes the function of the liver, helps with digestion and helps to spread the Qi. Green tea is healthier than black tea. It also has half of the caffeine. Drink at least one cup of green tea a day. All Chinese martial artists and Qigong masters drink tea regularly. It's recommended to drink tea at the end of your Qigong or Tai Chi practice. Green tea should be served at a lower temperature. Do not use boiling water for brewing, only use medium to hot water for loose green tea or for green tea bags.

  The benefits you will get from green tea depend on the quality, and how and where it was made.[19]
  The best green teas in the world are made in Japan. So look for a green tea with a label "made in Japan."

- Drink more water!!! Sometimes our bodies often mistake hunger for thirst. Try to drink as much water as you can. You need to understand that every function of our bodies depends on the proficient flow of water. It will keep you hydrated and alert. Also in Chinese Medicine it's not recommended to drink cold water, especially when it's cold outside.

  Keep water handy. Put water in front of you. I recommend spreading glasses of water throughout the house. Keep a bottle of water in the car and on your desk. That way water is always available to you. Tea and coffee do not count as water and can have the opposite effect and sometime can lead to dehydration.

Flavoring your Food

Chinese Medicine usually discusses five major flavors: salty, sour, sweet, bitter and pungent. Each flavor relates to an organ and has a certain effect on our health. In Chinese Medicine it's recommended to combine these flavors while you are cooking. That is the way you find the famous dishes in Chinese restaurants such as sweet and sour. The key is not too much or too little of any flavor.

---

[19] Tom Standage. *A History of the World in 6 Glasses*. New York: Walker and Company, 2005.

From the eastern medicine, food should always be balanced between warm (yang) and cold (yin).

Exercise in Nature

If weather permits try doing Qigong, Tai Chi, or any other physical activity outdoors and try to draw in nature's energy and relaxation. This is even better if you are surrounded by trees or next to a body of water. Exercising outside has a calming effect both emotionally and physically.

Try Walking More

Walking is the most basic and simple form of exercise and we all need to do more of it. Walking has a lot of benefits similar to jogging. Walking brings oxygen to the blood and every cell in the body. It also improves circulation, fights depression, helps with weight loss, lowers blood pressure and it's good for mental and emotional balance.

In modern times many people take cars and buses and don't get to enjoy the benefits of walking. They made their lives too convenient. In order to walk more, try to take the stairs instead of the elevator. Park the car five minutes away from your destination or get off the bus one station away and walk. Try to challenge yourself to be more active each day.

10 Minute Self Massage

This 10 minute self massage is based on Chinese medical theory. This method is very gentle and simple. The idea behind it is creating better Qi and blood circulation in the body. This massage can be done any time of the day and it's great just before sleep. You can do it by yourself or have your partner do it to you.
The massage covers several parts of the body:

1. **Massage the face**

Brush your hands together, then cover the face with the hands and rub your face up and down. Now place your palms close to the forehead, and move them downward along the sides of the nose to the lower jaw while rubbing. Massaging your temples is good for migraines. Finally, gently pull the ear lobes outwards with the thumb and the forefinger.

2. **Massage the neck and shoulders**

Slowly and gently massage the neck with the index and middle finger. Gently but firmly work your fingers in small circles, starting at the base of your skull and working down towards the shoulders. Try to keep the shoulders down and relaxed.

3. **Massage the shoulder**

Grip the shoulder muscles with fingers and the back of the hand and massage into the tender areas, moving down the shoulder. Hold your right arm straight in front of you. Gently massage your left palm down the whole length of your right arm. Repeat on the opposite side.

4. **Massage the legs**

Sit on the floor and stretch the legs straight. Massage the legs with both hands from the hip joints to the feet. Start with light motions and then dig in with your palm, moving in firmer circles.

5. **Massage the sole of the foot (bubbling spring)**

Dig your thumbs in a circular motion into the soles of your feet and the bottoms of your toes. Massage the soles of your feet either by creating circular motions with both of your thumbs, or putting your hand into a fist and running it up and down the soles of your feet.

Practice Everyday

Set up a regular schedule for your practice. As Master CK Chu writes: "Make the appointment with yourself, for yourself. ...Quiet often it is only the first few minutes that are less comfortable. Once the body gets involved, the mind follows."[20]

Balance

Balance is a challenge as we get older. One of the best health benefits of Qigong and Tai Chi is better balance! Practice inner balance by standing on one foot whenever you can. Try standing on one foot when you put your clothes or shoes. Also practice Golden Rooster Stands on One Leg Exercise.

Arms and Joints

The joints and the arms are very important. Rotate your arms, your shoulders and your legs at the hips through their full range of movement daily. This will help you avoid any injury.

Take it Easy

- Try to find the things that make you happy.

- Keep a regular schedule for work and rest.

- During your commute to work, on the subway or waiting in the post office, if you feel stress is coming, practice deep breathing. Tell yourself, "I am not in a rush."

- Try to find a few minutes during the day for a mini Qigong workout. Every day pick two different movements. Again, most of the movements only require a small space and can be done in a small office space.

---

[20] CK Chu. *The Book of Nei Kung*, New York: Sunflower Press, 2007. P, 29.

- If you feel somebody or a certain situation is making you stressful, take a mini break and do the full body shaking movement.

- Take a power nap.[21] A mid day nap is great for recharging the body. A power nap is anywhere between 10 to 30 minutes. Even a short five minute nap can have tremendous benefits, such as more energy to the entire body and focus. You can use an alarm clock to make sure you don't over sleep.

- Try to smile and laugh and, as the Eagles say, "Take it easy!"

---

[21] James B Mass. *Miracle Sleep Cure: The Key to a Long Life of Peak Performance.* London: Thorsons, 1998.

Glossary of Qigong Terms

Active Qigong (dong gong) – Qigong exercises that include movements.

Bagua – Literally "eight division." Also called eight trigrams.

Dantian – "Elixir Field." The center of gravity, breathing and energy located three inches below the navel.

Dao – The way of harmony within oneself, with others and nature.

Dao Yin – The most common ancient name for Qigong, means leading and guiding the Qi.

Dian – "To point" or "to press."

Eight Pieces of Brocade (Ba Dua Jin) – One of the most popular Qigong forms.

Five Elements – Five interacting energies that are most balanced for health, consisting of Wood, Fire, Earth, Metal and Water.

Fa Jin – the ability or skill to discharge explosive power in the form of a powerful blow.

Feng – "To seal" or "to cover."

Gua (Trigram) – Eight symbols which make up Daoist Bagua theory. They represent the fundamental principles of reality.

Horse Stance – The basic stance for Qigong and most martial arts.

Jin (Ching) – Strength, power, or expression of strength.

Kung Fu (Gongfu) – Gong means energy or work. Gongfu means "energy-time," anything that takes time and energy to learn is called Gongfu.

Kwa – The hip point, the key point when practicing Tai Chi.

Laozi – The original Daoist who wrote the *Daodejing*.

Le – Joy or happiness.

Ma Bu – Horse stance, one of the basic stances in Qigong and Chinese martial arts.

Meridians (Jing Mai) – The network of channels through which Qi is distributed and circulates.

Ming – the journey from life to death.

Neigong – Internal Kung fu.

Qi – Life energy, vital energy, breath of life, force, power, air.

Ren – Man or mankind.

Ren Qi – Hunan Qi.

San Cai – Three powers: Heaven, Earth and Man.

Sinking the Qi – Using your breath to help relax and calm the mind and body.

Shen – Spirit or spiritual energy. According to Chinese teachings, the Shen resides at the upper Dantian (the third eye).

Sung – Active relaxation. The process of removing tension from the body or the awareness of the body until tension can be dissolved.

Tai Chi Chuan – A Chinese internal martial arts based on the theory of Tai Chi (Grand Ultimatum). It's this force which creates two poles, Yin and Yang.

Wu Wei (woo'-way') – "No action," "no strain"; doing things naturally and effortlessness.

Wuji (Wu Chi) - No extreme. Wuji gave birth to yin and yang division.

Yang – the active aspect of reality that expresses itself in speech, light and heat.

Yi – mind, intention, idea. The mind in Qigong training is able to make you calm, peaceful and wise. The Yi leads or directs the Qi. Without Yi there is no Qi movement.

Yin – the receptive aspect of the universe that expresses itself in silence, darkness, coolness, and rest.

Bibliography

Bluestein, Jonathan. *Research of Martial Arts*, Create Space Independent Publishing Platform, 2014.

Cannon, Walter. *Bodily Changes in Pain, Hunger, Fear, and Rage.* New York: Appleton-Century-Crofts. *1929.*

Chen, Mark. *Old Frame Chen Family*, Berkley: Blue Snake Books, 2004.

Chia, Mantak. *Awaking Healing Energy Through the Tao*, Santa Fe, NH: Aurora Press, 1983.

Chris Jarmey. *The Theory and Practice of Taiji Qigong.* Berkley: North Atlantic Books, 2005.

Cohen, Kenneth S. *The Way of Qigong.* Toronto: Ballantine, 1997.

Chu, CK. *The Book of Nei Kung*, New York: Sunflower Press, 2007.

Elinwood Ellae. *Qigong the Basics, (Tuttle Martial Arts Basics),* Boston: Tuttle Publishing, 2004.

Frantzis, Bruce. *The Power of Internal Martial Arts and Chi: Combat and Energy Secrets of Ba Gua, Tai Chi and Hsing-I*, Berkeley: Blue Snake Books. 2007.

Frantzis, Bruce. *Opening the Energy Gates of Your Body*, Berkeley: Blue Snake Books. 2007.

Keay, John. *China: A History*, New York: Basic Books, 2011

Kohn, Livia. *Daoism and Chinese Culture*, Cambridge, MA: Three Pines Press, 2001.

Kristin Kupfer. Emergence and Development of Spiritual Religious Groups in the People's Republic of China after 1978 Dissertation.

Lee, Bruce. *Tao of Jeet Kune Do*. Santa Clarita: Ohara Publication, Inc, 1994.

Masaru Takahashi & Stephen Brown. *Qigong for Health: Chinese Traditional Exercise for Cure and Prevention*. Japan Publications, 1986.

Maas, James B. *Miracle Sleep Cure: The Key to a Long Life of Peak Performance*. London: Thorsons, 1998.

Mitchell, Damo. *Daoist Nei Gong: The Philosophical Art of Change*, London: Singing Dragon, 2011.

Palmer, David A. *Qigong Fever: Body, Science and Utopia in China*, New York: Columbia University Press, 2007.

Plaugher, Noel. *Standing Qigong for Health and Martial Arts*, Philadelphia: Singing Dragon, 2015

Qingie, Zhou. *10-Minute Primer Qigong*, London: Singing Dragon, 2009.

Standage, Tom. *A History of the World in 6 Glasses*, New York: Walker and Company, 2005.

Starr, Philip. *Developing Jin: Silk Reeling in Tai Chi and Internal Martial Arts*, Berkeley: Singing Dragon, 2014

Stone, Gene. *The Secrets of People Who Never Get Sick*, New York: Workman Publishing Company, 2010.

Wilson, Stanley. *Qigong for Beginners*, New York: Sterling Publishing, 1997

Yang, Jwing-Ming. *Eight Simple Qigong*. Massachusetts: YMAA Publication Center, 1997.

Yang, Jwing-Ming. *The Root of Chinese Chi Kung: The Secrets of Chi Kung Training,*. Massachusetts: YMAA Publication Center, 1989.

Yu, Yong Nian, *Zhan Zhuang: The Art of Nourishing Life*, Create Space Independent Publishing Platform; 1 edition, 2015.

Zeng, Qingnan. *Qigong and Chinese Self-Massage for Everyday Health Care*, Philadelphia: Singing Dragon, 2014.

Qigong Videos

Cohen, Ken. *Qigong: Traditional Chinese Exercises for Healing, Body, Mind and Spirit*, Sounds True, Inc., 1996.

Cohen, Matthew. *Qigong Fire and Water*, Acacia, 2007.

Garripoli Francesco and Garripoli Daisy Lee, *Qigong for Beginners*, Gaiam, 2004.

Garripoli Francesco and Garripoli Daisy Lee, *Qigong for Stress Relief*, Gaiam, 2008.

Holden, Lee. Qi *Workout Am/Pm*, Sound True Inc., 2010.

O'Shea, Lisa. *Qigong for Women*, YMAA, 2012.

Pai, Chris. *Qigong for Beginners*, Body Wisdom, 2009.

Yang, Jwing-Ming. *Five Animal Sports Qigong*, YMAA, 2008.

Yang, Jwing-Ming. *Simple Qigong: Exercises for Health - The Eight Pieces of Brocade*, YMAA, 2003.

Printed in Great Britain
by Amazon